REFLECTIONS
OF A
PSYCHIATRIST

REFLECTIONS OF A PSYCHIATRIST

OF A

PSYCHIATRIST

A Journey of Five Decades

SHAILJA CHATURVEDI

Library of Congress Control Number: 2020923155
ISBN: Hardcover   978-1-6641-0223-1
                  Softcover   978-1-6641-0222-4
                  eBook   978-1-6641-0221-7

Print information available on the last page.

Rev. date: 06/02/2021

To order additional copies of this book, contact:
Xlibris
AU TFN: 1 800 844 927 (Toll Free inside Australia)
AU Local: 0283 108 187 (+61 2 8310 8187 from outside Australia)
www.Xlibris.com.au
Orders@Xlibris.com.au
820568

Dedicated to my mentor, my inspiration,
The man who believed in me

My father Dr MP Chaturvedi (1918-1979)

CONTENTS

ACKNOWLEDGEMENT

This is the story of an endless journey, without a destination. The incredible journey of privilege: which restored my faith and confidence, in the profoundness of human relationships. Sharing other people's most private and painful experiences, with their unconditional trust in me, was the most humbling, educational, fulfilling and rewarding experience of my life. It was the ultimate measure of my success as a psychiatrist.

I experienced devastating failures, and resounding success, both professionally and personally, as part of this journey, which indeed made me a better and more resilient person.

I never ceased to be amazed by the capacity for love, courage, endurance, forgiveness and resilience, of ordinary people, which often gets eclipsed, by the mental illness.

My patients have been my most important teachers, who taught me about love, life, courage and resilience. I am eternally grateful to them for grooming me, from a carefree, naïve, young woman into a mature, compassionate and well grounded professional.

I owe so much to my parents, who together gave me the most secure and stable start, in life, instilling hope, aspiration and confidence for acceleration, and success.

I am extremely grateful to Prof Gin Malhi who was kind enough to read the book, make constructive commenrts and write such a complimentary foreword.

Family support is inevitable, in accomplishing a task like writing a book. I am grateful to my family for their support, and inspiration in their own way.

The knowledge and wisdom I gained, over the past nearly 5 decades: professionally growing, within the culture and academia of Australian psychiatry, has been boundless, which I have endeavored, to precisely reiterate as the moral of the story, learnt over a lifetime, in this book. For this I must thank, the editors and the authors of ANZJP and Australasian psychiatry, for its vast literature, from where most of my references and reading has generated.

I must also thank the publisher specially Cherry Noel for her patience and guidance

I may not have accomplished all I wished and planned, the day I entered the medical school in 1962, but enough not to be disappointed.

FOREWORD

Title Reflections of a psychiatrist

This book is unusual for several reasons. Firstly, it only has a single author, which is uncommon for such a comprehensive text. Secondly, the author is a woman, and an Indian woman at that, who draws on her experiences of psychiatry in Australia. On top of this, as if this wasn't already enough to set the book apart, its content is an amalgam of history, facts and personal reflections. As a consequence, it has something for everyone. However, this should not be taken to mean that the book is in anyway disjointed. Indeed, one of the most endearing aspects of the text is that throughout it tells a story.

For those wanting to understand how psychiatry has evolved in Australia in recent decades, the text provides an overview of notable institutions, legislative developments, and the many significant changes that have occurred in our understanding and conceptualisation of psychiatry. Younger psychiatrists would have heard about mental hospitals such as Bloomsfield, Callan Park, and Gladesville, and the many associated tales. However, in *Reflections of a Psychiatrist*, we hear a personal account of someone who has lived and worked in these places as part of her training. Someone who knows the patients and their families, Shailja provides a personal account of the history of these hospitals, enriched by her own observations and views. She describes for example how picturesque the hospitals were – *"The sprawling grounds, beautifully flowering gardens, ... and my own little nearly 100 years old cottage"* – few (if any) hospitals of the modern era will be remembered with such fondness.

In addition to providing history and context, the book also walks us through the majority of the major psychiatric disorders and provides a broad, clinically relevant overview. Given the easy access to facts and figures, the book preoccupies itself with key and interesting aspects of each disorder, noting for example points of contention, and those that over the years have been of particular interest, either because of changes in classification or treatment. The net result is that the book is easy to read, and the information it provides is readily assimilated. Its readability in these sections of the book, means that it would serve as a good primer for anyone interested in getting an overview of psychiatry, particularly in the Australian context, without having to be overwhelmed by epidemiological data, detailed pathophysiology or complex pharmacology.

Throughout the book, there is an ever-present sense of the author, and the fact that she is taking us on a journey – a road that she has travelled – and that we are sharing in her observations and the thoughts that these have invoked. Snippets of personal opinion and perspective bring the text to life and imbue the words with emotional qualities. When reading the book, it is clear that the person speaking to you, who's voice you can hear internally, is speaking from experience. It's someone who has indeed reflected on the subject for many years, thought about people and their lives, and how mental illness has impacted them deeply and truly.

The structure of the book is straightforward, with 32 chapters and its clear organisation allows the reader to pick up the story at any point. Many sections are mini stories in themselves that can be read standalone, but to truly and fully appreciate the book, it is perhaps best read from the beginning.

Amazingly, the book also covers a broad range of topics that one wouldn't normally expect to see in a psychiatric text, reflecting perhaps the breadth of knowledge, interest and experience of the author. Topics such as technology, and the development of tools in digital health, this sits alongside circadian science – a useful introduction into the importance of this theme within psychiatry. But Shailja also extends herself further, commenting on the ecosystem, climate change and the responsibilities of psychiatrists with respect to these global issues. Closer to home and more central to our experiences, Shailja delves briefly into spirituality, drawing connections between Indian philosophy and psychotherapeutic techniques. But she does not stop here. Importantly, the book mentions the ethics of psychiatry in relation to the obligations of our profession and this then links to another couple of important sections within the book that highlight the plight of refugees and our international responsibilities.

In addition to adding further interest, these sections of the book truly make it essential reading. This is especially the case because Shailja also does not limit herself to just the mind and its many facets. Instead, she also discusses physical health, noting its importance and its links to mental health. This is captured by consultation liaison psychiatry, perhaps the specialty of most interest to trainee psychiatrists of today. But those aspects that are less popular, and perhaps waning in terms of interest, are also given a boost, such as academic psychiatry. For example, in this section, Shailja – drawing on her own experiences – attempts to impress the importance of maintaining research and education at the heart of psychiatry and clinical practice.

As you are probably now beginning to realise, the territory covered by the book is vast, albeit many topics are only considered briefly. But Shailja does not relent and the journey continues to the medical-legal interface of psychiatry, with a detailed discussion of the medical board, which is made all the more interesting by dissection of real-world cases. Collectively, these and some previous sections, provide a nice foundation for more philosophical considerations such as human rights, euthanasia, and the complex challenges facing forensic psychiatry.

It is easy to write a safe text, stick to the topics that are well established, impart facts and synthesise information, and whilst some of this is necessary, it usually culminates in an uninteresting text that is rarely memorable. There are many facts and figures in this book, along with descriptions and definitions, but the main value is captured in the title – the reflections. It is the impressions, the personal account, the individual perspective, that this book provides, that is most fascinating. The only fact of importance is that it covers an enormous number of topics, and embraces issues that are contentious and thought provoking. For example, Shailja does not shy away form the mental health of doctors, an issue we are all aware of but seldom wish to discuss. She also highlights the current controversies within gender dysphoria by detailing an interesting case study, an approach that makes the book much more relatable and clinically relevant. This is a particular strength of the book, and she has used case studies to good effect throughout, to illustrate the vagaries of various disorders.

In sum, Dr. Chaturvedi, Shailja, has provided an invaluable set of insights, shared her thinking and her views, educated us about psychiatry in an Australian context and enriched us while doing so. It's a book that I heartily recommend that you read, and then, reflect.

Prof Gin Malhi
Professor of Psychiatry University of Sydney
Editor in Chief Australian NewZealand Journal of Psychiatry
Chief Investigator NHMRC Program Grant
Editor in Chief international journal Acta Neuropsychiatrica
Scientific Advisory Board international Bipolar Foundation

INTRODUCTION

"With half a laugh of hearty zest, I strip me off my coat and vest.
Then heeding not the frigid air
I fling away my underwear.
So having nothing else to doff,
I rip my epidermis off,
More secrets to acquaint you with, I pare my bones to strips of pith
And when the expose is done I hang, a cog-web skeleton.
While you sit there: aloof, remote, and, will not shed your overcoat."

The purpose of writing this book is: the recapitulation of the wisdom and knowledge I acquired, both professionally and personally, over the past 5 decades of journey in the pursuit of, perfection.

Psychiatry was not my choice for post graduation, with almost nil background in the field: hardly uncovering its mystique. The limited opportunities, for an international medical graduate in Australia, was indeed a blessing for me to compromise, with the availability, once I got my registration and completed the residency. Reflecting on it, after nearly 5 decades, the journey has not only made a profound impact on all aspects of my life, but has been one of the most uplifting experiences of unrelenting privilege, passion and fascination.

It seemed like, early days for psychiatry, not only in my homeland, but also in Australia, when it was still establishing its credibility; from being on the lighter side of the serious business of medicine: akin to entertainment.

The upheaval and the changes of early 1970s were exciting, daunting, and challenging. White Australia Policy was repealed, which allowed influx of Indian doctors like myself, and the troops from Vietnam War, were finally returning home after a decade. And, an internationally commendable book of an Australian author Germaine Greer 'The Female Eunuch' was causing ripples, challenging the conservative and sexually inhibited young women raised in 1940s and 50s. Women's rights movement was roaring in the voice of the Australian singer Helen Reddy 'I Am a Woman', the first Australian singer to top the US chart.

It was the year after when 'Sybil-Account of Multiple Personality Disorder' (Disassociated Identity Disorder DID) was published, by Flora Rheta Schrieber, only to be discredited later, (Borch-Jacobson) by the publication of Sybil Exposed, revealing the deception of patient, psychiatrist and the journalist (Nathan D 2011).

I walked through the epidemic of Munchausen Syndrome, False Memory Syndrome, and Satanic-Ritual Abuse, not to mention the oedipal-complex and even homosexuality, defined as sexually deviant personality disorder, needing aversive therapy. The corner was turned, when Australian and American Medical Associations removed it from their list of illnesses and disorders, in 1973. It is interesting that now homosexuality is an accepted life style and non-acceptance is homophobia. A civil rights milestone Mardi Grass was born, in the midst of the protests, clashes and arrests in 1978.

As psychiatry was attempting to come out of its dungeon: the decaying neglect of mental hospitals, and the zeitgeist of antipsychiatry, there was no dearth of people trying to sabotage. The Church of Scientology continued its attack on psychiatry, specially concerning deep sleep therapy, ECT, psychosurgery and involuntary hospitalisations.

Prominent in the anti psychiatry movement was: Thomas Szasz a reputable academic psychiatrist and psychoanalyst, from New York. Of his many publications 'Myth of Mental Illness', 'Psychiatry The Science of Lies' and 'Manufacturing Mental Illness' did the most damage.

In 1974 Martin Roth the main author of authoritative text-book Clinical Psychiatry and the President of Royal College of Psychiatrist, engaged in a debate with Szasz, which was published in British Journal of Psychiatry (Roth M 1976). This had a significant role in restoring the confidence, in the validity of psychiatry, and its pivotal role in general medicine.

The mystery, the enigma and the curiosity made psychiatry even more adventurous than other fields of medicine. Interestingly psychiatry has phases of heightened concepts, over-extending the mandate of medicine, which makes it vulnerable to legal and social manipulations. Therefore self-diagnosed patients, with their superficial knowledge, started weighing up its use, as protection, to justify their dysfunction.

References

Borch-Jacobson M and Herbert Spiegel. NYRB, 24 April 1997 Sybil-The Making of a Disease: An interview with Dr Herbert Spiegel.

Nathan D. Sybil Exposed: The Extraordinary Story Behind the Famous Multiple Personality Case. New York: Simon and Schuster.

Roth M. Schizophrenia and theories: of Thomas Szasz. British Journal of Psychiatry 1976 129: 317-326.

Contemporary Australian Psychiatry

The controversies which drew social and political attention, fortunately forced psychiatry to review, its practices, in favor of transparency, The confinement of mentally ill patients, a vestige of British colonial history, was the obvious next challenge, needing reforms in the area. This led to patient's rights in the modes of treatment, including psychosurgery, deep sleep therapy and ECT (unmodified). In mid 1980s the Royal Commission started investigating, the controversial practice of leucotomy, which led, to the catastrophe of Chelmsford, a private psychiatric hospital in Sydney with tragic consequences for both: the psychiatrists and the patients.

I was fascinated to read the Reception House admission notes, of long stay psychiatric patients, dating back to early last century as 'insane', 'imbecile' and 'lunatic' to describe the mentally ill.

Deinstitutionalisation

It commenced in mid seventies, closing the large mental hospitals with patient numbers of around 2000, and relocating patients into smaller general hospital psychiatric units. It was a vital change from the hospital settings of lush green rural sprawl, to a, large and crowded, city hospitals. Fortunately with the experience of transition, there was more appreciation of environment and mental health. It also provided insight into the coercive, paternalistic and bland site of hospital setting.

It is well known, that physical environment including wise planning of hospital space, has the potential, to impact upon healing, as well as lessening of conflicts. Hippocrates referred to the environment as an important factor for healing. The newer psychiatric units are focused on, patient centered model of care and recovery. Less institutional, more homely, holistic and aesthetic environment, were important factors in designing these mental health facilities (Golembiewski JA. 2015). This has led to the concept of Nidotherapy. Derived from Latin word nidus, meaning a nest. It is classed as psychotherapy, though instead of changing the patient, it changes the environment, which includes social, physical and personal space (Spencer et al 2010). It is something we all do to manipulate our environment for the best fit and for optimal functioning. This must be an important consideration in comprehensive patient management.

Advances in psychiatry; from late 1970s gradually eclipsed, the long tradition of Freudian psychoanalysis, which had argued, that most mental disorders were caused by, emotional and sexual conflicts. During my working life, medical science in psychiatry has advanced dramatically.

Towards the close of last century, psychiatry appeared to be marching with confidence, having addressed many of its controversial closets. It opened up the floodgates of evidence-based medicine, and embraced the bio-psychosocial model of mental illness.

It has indeed been an exciting period, though not without challenges. More than any other branch of medicine, psychiatry is the product of its society and culture in which it emerges and evolves, which inculcates wider view of an illness, in training a psychiatrist. Modern psychiatry has helped other fields of medicine in humanising and de-medicalising, human adversities, distress and clinical helplessness, amenable to positive relationships, environment, communication, compassion and understanding.

There are three main influences which affect individual's well being: genetic, life circumstances and involvement in active pursuits and special interests. Genetic factors interacting with upbringing and environment, account for 50% variation in people. Although poverty is a significant contributor, of unhappiness and an obstacle to wellbeing, increase in income above the poverty line, fails to proportionately alter life satisfaction (Easterline R. 2003).

So what has motivated me, to delve into reflecting on my professional journey, and sharing it with you, the reader? Is it the fact that psychiatry is the most comprehensive and encompassing branch of medicine? Psychiatry is so relevant to the real life, of an ordinary person, yet it is also at the forefront of the scientific world. Deinstitutionalisation has been the most significant factor, in the growth of this long neglected vital medical specialty.

Apart from psychiatry's closeness to an ideal life and human psych, the brain and the mind are valued the most, of any human organ. And yet psychiatry has been an undervalued and controversial branch of medicine. Despite its unprecedented development in the clinical sciences, psychiatry still remains a poor cousin in the medical domain because of its diagnostic instability. Phenomenology rather than patho-physiology, remains the stronghold of its trajectory, with significant impact of socio-psycho environmental factors. The dimensional nature of psychiatric diagnosis makes it look like, a pathological extension of acceptable human behavior, devoid of any definite biomarker. Psychiatric disorders are syndromes rather than an illness. It has a long way to go, in its enthusiastic search of psychiatric labels, and mental health literacy, which often results in over diagnosis (Malhi G, et al 2020).

Unfortunately despite its excellent academic and research progress, psychiatry falls short of proving a clinical success

References

Easterline R. Explaining Happiness. Proceedings of National Academy of Science, Washington DC 2003; 100:11176-11183.

Golembiewski JA. Mental health facility design: The case for person-centered care. ANZJP 2015, 49: (3) 203-206.

Malhi G, et al. ANZJP 2020 54(3) 324-328.

Spencer S J, Rutter D, et al. (2010) Integration of nidotherapy in the management of mental illness and antisocial personality: A qualitative study. International Journal of Social Psychiatry 56: 50-59.

MENTAL HEALTH

Definition

THE CONSTITUTION OF World Health Organisation states, that the absence of mental disorder: is not the sufficient condition for mental health. Instead, mental health is the state of well being; that is determined by social, psychological and biological factors, which together enable the individual to realise their abilities, cope with the normal life stresses, work productively and contribute to their communities (www.who.int/media /factsheets/fs220/en).

Do we take mental health for granted? Of course, we do, as the natural course of life. And we do so to a large extent. One thing which has impressed me from my experiences with people: with or without mental illness; is that, each of us has an inbuilt human resource, that no matter how desperate, their situations may appear from outside, people have pockets of exceptional strength, resilience, creativity and innovation. Therefore unnecessary or sometimes contradictory help must be avoided. One cannot underestimate human potential and determination.

Intentional activities and active engagement, can account for 40 percent of people's variations in happiness. Life satisfaction, personal development and social wellbeing with altruistic thinking, appear most significant in influencing wellbeing (Mark N and Shah H 2005).

Subjective wellbeing, though personal, is a strong measure of mental health, which includes cognitive component, evaluating satisfaction with life, and an affective component, involving positive affect.

Subjective wellbeing improves with increasing income though plateaus after a higher level (Mulder RT, et al. 2020).

Poverty remains one of the biggest global health problems, compromising socioeconomic and child development, and the future of the world. This is not necessarily the description of the 3rd. world countries, but affluent Western countries like Australia, also have their fair share, largely limited to its Indigenous population.

During my nearly five decades in the field, the impact of mental health on life, has been increasingly recognized and psychiatry has begun, gaining its well overdue credit, as the foundation for wellbeing, and effective functioning of an individual. Therefore psychiatry must become the most comprehensive branch of medicine, determined by a range of interrelated factors like physical, social, psychological, cultural and spiritual. Nevertheless mental illness is the most significant driver of; years lived with disability (YLDs) comparable to cardiovascular and circulatory diseases, in terms of its impact on disability adjusted life years (DALYs) (Vigo D, et al. 2016).

Like any other country Australia is endeavoring to provide the best possible mental health services to its nationals. In its latest report, Productivity Commission of Australia has acknowledged that reforms of mental health system would produce, large benefits. Improvement in people's quality of life is valued, up to $18 billions annually, with additional benefit of $1.3 billions annually, due to increased economic participation. By investing, up to $2.4 billions on the identified priority reforms, benefits of about $ 17 billions can be achieved, generating savings of up to $ 1.2 billion per year (Australian Gov.).

References

Australian Government Productivity Commission Mental Health enquiry-Report 2020.

Mark N, Shah H. A well-being manifesto for a flourishing Society, Journal of Mental Health Promotion2005; 3,4:9-15.

Mulder RT, Scott KM, et al. Making sense of vulnerability paradox in cross-national studies of mental disorders: Lessons from research on subjective Well-being. ANZJP 2020. Vol. 54 (7) 664-666.

Vigo D, Thornicroft G, et al. 2016 Estimating the true global burden of mental illness, The Lancet psychiatry 3: 171-178.

MENTAL HOSPITALS

MY PSYCHIATRY TRAINING was within the long stay mental institutions of NSW, often referred to as "asylum" or "funny farms", and dreaded by general public. Therefore these hospitals were built away from public access, even if these were within the city limits. The history of care, of mentally deranged people, who were either misfit or socially incompatible, goes back to medieval era. It has travelled through the complex road of changing philosophies of the time: from cruelty, to rejection, to compassion until finally mental health issues became recognised and elevated to illnesses, as variation of human diseases. The asylums, created to segregate mentally ill individuals from the community, with intention of providing special attention and care, were proliferating around the world for more than a millennium. However Australia as a British colony; only started to think of containing its "lunatics" and "idiots" in 1810 when its population had grown to 11,566."

History

Castle Hill asylum in 1811 followed by Liverpool asylum in 1825, were established for this purpose of containment. Both of these facilities were far from ideal, even for those times.

They were mostly staffed by non-medical personnel, and bonded convicts. These institutions were subsequently replaced by Tarban Creek Asylum in 1838, the purpose built mental hospital, with appointment of Joseph Thomas Digby, as its superintendent and his wife, as the matron arriving from England. Digby was not a medical practitioner, but was likely appointed due to his experience in British asylums. Following many complaints about his management of patients, Dr Campbell replaced him till the arrival of Dr Fred Norton Manning in 1867.

Gladesville Hospital

I was privileged to have worked in the building, which was occupied by the superintendent of Tarban Creek Asylum and had been renamed Gladesville Hospital by the time of my tenure there. NSW Mental Health Review Tribunal office was fortunate to lease this grand home. My fondness for mentally ill people warmed up many folds, as I walked on the grounds, once occupied by the people, who gave me my profession and meaning in life. It still pleases me to see the streets and the buildings in and around the hospital, named after the distinguished innovators, who laid the foundation bricks for the care of mentally ill.

Bloomfield Hospital

Emotions aside, my first experience with a psychiatric patients, was in early 1970s, when as a trainee psychiatrist I joined the staff of Bloomfield hospital in Orange; built in 1923, some three hundred kilometer from Sydney. The sprawling grounds, beautifully flowering gardens, the immaculate golf club, the old well restored buildings, the historic landscape, and my own little nearly hundred-year-old cottage: all won my heart at the first sight. Remaining there for a year, I learnt that the journey into reforming the care for mentally ill was just beginning. The criteria for admission was much more wider than could be accepted within the modern definition of mental illness. There was a separate Inebriates Ward to accommodate monthly arrival of busloads of people from city hospitals under the Inebriates Act, who were sent to Bloomfield to remove them from the source of alcohol. These patients saved their pension for 3 months, relapsed after their discharge, and returned again for the cycle of 3 months to restore their alcohol damaged body. There were patients who had lived in the hospital, for up to, nearly five decades having been transferred from city hospitals. The patients and their families both found hospital a better alternative to home. There were patients who had difficult personality (not mental illness), or impaired intelligence, whose behaviour would have been intolerable in the community. There would have been overcrowding, with nearly 1600 inpatients, but for the vast open spaces, and many daily facilities, which indeed needed improvement. There was accepted and deeply entrenched, widespread culture, not only in Bloomfield, but throughout the state run psychiatric institutions, where nursing staff occupied strong informal position of authority backed by their unions. Any change in the long tradition of custodial care, and the management, was unwelcome. Patients seemed the least important subject, in the complex hierarchy.

Nevertheless the rehabilitation programs, kept most of them occupied with hospital maintenance services, like gardening, kitchen, laundry and other housekeeping activities, which has sadly disappeared from the modern psychiatric units.

Bloomfield being the only state hospital in Western NSW, covered large number of country towns past Blue Mountains, till the state border. It provided outpatients services to all of its catchment areas. This also gave me the opportunity, to learn about the real culture of my adopted country, which was still grappling with the concept of new Australians like myself. I was once asked, if I was of aboriginal descent. Bewildered by the question, I foolishly said as how many aboriginal doctors, the person had seen. My only experience at the time with Australian aboriginal group was: the few patients and their families I met through my work. At another time coming back from our clinic in Lightening Ridge, a small outback town in the North-Western NSW: the world renowned center, of the mining of opal gemstones, we stopped for lunch at the RSL club. My colleague asked me to wait in the car. I was later surprised to find out, that he needed special permission, for my entry to the club as a non-white female, though White Australia policy was no longer operational.

Parramatta Psychiatric Centre

My next training post for another year was at North Parramatta Psychiatric Centre. A hospital with history, heritage and legacy; compounded my long-standing interest in history. The location of the current hospital, was chosen by, Governor Lachlan Macquarie on a 4 acres block, along Parramatta River in 1818, for the 1st purpose built, Female Factory in the colony, and model for others, in the country. It was built by Francis Greenway the first government architect of the colony who was transported to Australia for the crime of forgery in 1814 at the age of 37 years. Over the next 2 decades before his death, Greenway designed some of the finest buildings in Australia, including Hyde Park Barracks, St James Church and Old Government House in Sydney, just to name a few.

The Female Factory was the home, for at least half of the convict women, sent as prisoners, to the colony of NSW, onwards from year 1821, accommodating 1203 women as well as children. It served as a place of assignments, hospital, a marriage bureau, a factory, an asylum and a prison for those, who committed a crime in the colony. The women manufactured cloth-linen and wool, did spinning, knitting, straw plating, washing, cleaning, rock breaking and oakum picking (twisted rope like material made from jute or hemp fibre). They were credited with the first manufactured export of the colony, in 1822: producing 55 meters of woven cloth.

The first industrial action in Australia took place in 1847, when the women of the Factory revolted against the poor condition and the reduced ration. The Factory subsequently closed down, giving way to the Convict Lunatics and the Invalid Asylum in 1849. The building described as unsightly and ruinous pile, was demolished and the new hospital building was completed in 1885.

Its current status as Institute of Psychiatry, since 1995 is the fitting tribute, to build a world of equal human rights, in an attempt to subdue the sufferings of, the women and their children over a century ago.

The present Cumberland hospital was renamed in 1983, having gone through its identity as a Mental Institution, Lunatic Asylum and North Parramatta Psychiatric Hospital.

In 1937 Parramatta Female Factory was the subject, of the film 'New Shores'.

It must have been an amazing journey of hardships and resilience, hard to comprehend for my generation, as I was trying to process, the unlimited depth of human emotions, the adversities of life-long impaired mind, and feelings of suffocation, for which I did not have an answer.

The Beatle mania was still alive and well, Hippy culture was the contemporary fashion, for the youngsters, and Elvis Presley had unrelenting queues of his admirers towards mid 70s. So what was common between them? Either inadvertently or misperceived apparent message, they conveyed was: condoning the use of mood elevating drugs to find happiness and peace.

In the charming garden setting of flowering Wisteria along side of the Parramatta River, the hospital enshrined its drug and alcohol ward, naming it **Wisteria House**. This was the culmination of untiring efforts, of the crusader Dr Stella Dalton AM to treat, heroin addiction with Methadone. In 1969 Stella became the first prescriber of methadone in Australia. She believed that methadone, replacing heroin, allowed its users to lead a reasonably happy, functional and normal life, though was not able to convince the NSW government, for funding the program. The legacy of Vietnam War, in early 70s, doubled the use of illicit drugs, which prompted government to approve seed funding, and she started the first inpatient detox unit in Wisteria House. I did my 6 months rotation with Stella: an elegant, well-spoken woman with compassion and dedication. She was convincing in the success of her mission, a good role model for a budding psychiatrist in me. Wisteria House was an egalitarian, democratic group like a therapeutic community of the time. They made their own rules, decided on admissions and support, or reprimand for breaking the rules, going to work either within or outside the hospital, contributing in housekeeping both financially and physically. The dedicated staff members were, available whenever required. I learnt a very big lesson, that given the trust and responsibility in a supportive environment of empathy and understanding: can bring out the desired change in many wayward personalities.

Callan Park

My last training halt was Callan Park. I perceived at the outset of my training, that unless I worked in Callan Park, I was not a real psychiatrist. Perhaps, because it was progressive, in the sense that it was the first hospital in NSW, admitting patients without committal, the first in Australia to establish Cerebral Surgery and Research Unit (1957) headed by an eminent psychiatrist Dr Harry Baily, and the first hospital to have laboratory, where studying the pathology of mental diseases in NSW began. So I was thrilled with the news of winning: my choice of the hospital. It was one of the most significant periods, both personally for me, and for the transformation of psychiatric services in NSW. The highlight for me was; entry to the College of Psychiatrist as a member, and for the hospital: it was the massive reform by shifting its long stay patients, into nearby boarding houses, and changing the infamous image of Callan Park, by renaming it; Rozelle Hospital, after the suburb where it was located, with amalgamation of adjoining Broughton Hall psychiatric clinic.

Broughton Hall: an army hospital of World-War 1 was converted as a day hospital in 1921. During my time, part of it housed child and adolescent unit under Dr Marie Bashir, (with whom I later worked as a part-time Mental Health Review Tribunal member), the Institute of Psychiatry and the living quarters for the hospital doctors

There is no end to the stories about Callan Park. One of which was; that there was an underground tunnel system, transporting unsightly patients from ship ports, to Callan Park facility, and then to Gladesville hospital. The intricate water tunnel system apparently stretched from Sydney Harbour to Callan park, and Gladesville hospital, to move patients underground to avoid infecting the citizens, and keep them out of the view. However it was never proven and has been disputed for years.

Living and working in Callan park, we enjoyed these, along with other ghost stories, like mysterious figures appearing in photographs and eerie feelings, when walking around certain wards at night.

The Hospital for The Insane was purpose built on 150 acre land, between 1880 and 1884, on the property by the same name Callan Park, independent of Gladesville hospital, to ease the overcrowding.

There have been increasing reports, of human rights violations in psychiatric institutions, and irregularities in their optimal care. Alongside was the scientific progress expanding the field of psychiatry.

More humane treatment of psychiatric patients, parallel to people with physical illnesses, as well as changing public perception, led to the birth of private psychiatric hospitals as well as planning to build psychiatric units in general hospitals. Late 1960s and early 1970s saw the trend, towards reducing institutional beds to fund, community and general hospital based care. So I was the part of the exodus program, finding suitable supervised accommodation in the community for the patients, who never experienced independent living, being street wise or basic life skills. To make the transition smooth they returned to hospital rehabilitation program or to the industrial unit to minimize the trauma with sense of abandonment.

My term in Callan Park gave me the opportunity to work in the Neuropsychiatric unit (old Cerebral Surgery and Research unit), a tertiary multi disciplinary service offering assessment and management of broad range of psychiatric, neurological and neurodegenerative disorders. My experience at NPI was later replicated in a survey of trainees who worked in Neuropsychiatry Unit at the Royal Melbourne Hospital between 1993 and 2017 (Thomas Rego, et al 2020). The feedback of this group was overwhelmingly positive. The sub-specialty rotation was highly valued in their career path with introduction to research and the wide variety of clinical presentations.

I also got an opportunity of working in the forensic ward.

For my dissertation, I chose to write a case of a patient, which intrigued me, as he killed both his parents. I wanted to dip through his mind for the reasons. His mother: he killed as she was nagging him to get a job. He soon after killed his father, whom he thought will not let him live in peace. Despite his mentally deranged mind, I could not conciliate with his reasoning. So I foolishly decided to probe further, which irritated him to no end, and he slapped hard on my face before walking out. I was shaken by this most unexpected reaction of my patient. I sat quietly and it took me at least 15 minutes before I could compose myself.

Although Callan Park was regarded as the finest mental hospital in the commonwealth, it may have been like the one eyed man, in the community of blinds. There were many reports and complaints, about sections of staff being incompetent, dishonest, delinquent and even sadistic, along with more general conditions of a mental hospital, whose obsolete system of locked ward had bred apathy, dirt and decadence. In 1950s there was overcrowding of well over 1500 patients including floridly psychotic, mentally retarded, epileptics, criminals and all other dysfunctional people: no one wanted. Some of the patients, who were reasonably well, and could have responded to timely appropriate treatment, also regressed in the hostile negative environment. The patient care was demeaning, and defied human dignity, with poor concept of hygiene. Patient abuse was common, in the name of controlling their unacceptable behaviour. The enquiry into the conditions at Callan Park conducted by Public Service Board in 1948, obviously failed to make any noticeable change. The hospital was trenchantly criticized in the past and the conditions were ripe for scandal.

Following a condemning article in Sydney Morning Herald in 1960 the government took a serious look at the repeated complaints of the disgruntled Medical Superintendent of Callan Park Dr Harry Baily. Decision was made for a judicial enquiry, with appointment of the Royal Commission for investigations, which began the following year. It disclosed the general deficiencies in the mental hospital system, which were, accepted in the past, but could not be overlooked by the contemporary social attitudes. Being in the position of power in NSW mental health, both the Director of State Psychiatric Services and the Medical Superintendent of Callan Park were held responsible for the abominable state of the hospital and were deposed as the result of it.

I joined NSW mental health services a decade after the report of the conclusion of Royal commission was released, though the grounding of its application was still palpable. It introduced the concept of preventive psychiatry, removing its isolation from general medical practice and hospitals. It emphasized the role of multidisciplinary team, like medical practitioners, paramedical professionals, nurses, clergymen, counselors and the frontline professional: advocating for their technical training. It expanded the residential care to outpatient and day hospital services, based in the community.

The other significant changes were in the area of disability, segregation of which, relieved the mental hospital crowding, and provided excellent service from prenatal diagnosis to the treatment, rehabilitation and residential care of mentally ill people.

In 1967 the Commonwealth Social Services Act was amended to grant the invalid pension to mentally retarded persons over the age of 16 years.

The Institute of Psychiatry

The Institute of Psychiatry was created in 1964, under its own Act of 1963 as statutory authority, per the recommendation of the Royal Commission, operating independently. Its status was not without fierce opposition from the Post-graduate Committee in Medicine of the Sydney University, wanting to integrate it with other postgraduate studies. The Institute also succeeded in replacing the long established Diploma in Psychological Medicine. Dr Maurice Sainsbury remained its director till his retirement. A highly respected humble man who related with such warmth with his trainees that it made each one of us feel so special. I later worked with him, as a part-time member of Mental Health review tribunal.

I was fortunate to have entered at the stage, when psychiatry was just turning the corner stepping out in the liberated, demonstrative, liberal and open world with recognition of human dignity and basic rights. Hearing the horrid stories of ECT without anaesthesia, I was relieved that in my era, it was modified with anaesthetics and muscle relaxants.

References

Thomas Rego, D Erante et al Trainee experience in a specialist neuropsychiatry training position Australasian Psychiatry 2020 Vol 2891 95-100.

SCHIZOPHRENIA

PSYCHIATRY HAS LARGELY remained a synonym of madness meaning schizophrenia.

So I need to start the book with this label.

The most significant, dreaded and most researched psychiatric diagnosis is: of schizophrenia, a heterogynous syndrome with lifetime prevalence of 1% associated with, high level of disability. It remains poorly understood, with current treatment less than ideal, and estimated rate of recovery 13.5% (Jaaskelainen E, et al. 2013).

Epidemiology and Risk factors

There is robust evidence to identify place of birth as a risk factor. Population based studies from Holland (Marcelis M, et al.1998) and Denmark found about 2.4% relative risk of developing schizophrenia, when born in metropolitan as compared to rural area (Mortensen PB, et al. 1999).

World Mental Health Survey of WHO (2008) on lifetime prevalence of mental illness revealed lower rate in low and middle-income countries against high-income countries, which came as a surprise (Scott, K M, et al 2008).

It is possible that cultural and lifestyle factors, like community and extended family engagement promote, the supportive network and acceptance.

Migrant status has been found with markedly increased risk for schizophrenia specially, for first and secondgenerations (Cantor-Graae E, et al. 2005).

Australian studies have found increased reporting of trauma in the background of psychiatric illnesses (Scott J, et al. 2007).

Prenatal nutrition has a significant effect on the fetus. During the World War 2, the well-documented Dutch hunger winter famine, produced offspring with increased risk for schizophrenia and schizophrenia spectrum personality disorders (Susser ES.et al.1992).

The risk of prenatal nutrition was further proven with starvation of catastrophic famine in China during the Cultural Revolution (St Clair D, et al.2005).

Vitamin D and maternal micronutrients like homocysteine (marker of folate metabolism) have been also implicated in the etiology of schizophrenia (Brown AS, et al. 2007).

Infections like influenza (Covid 19?), rubella, toxoplasma gondii and possibly herpes simplex virus type 2, may have adverse effect on the fetus in utero (Buka SL, et al. 2001).

Pregnancy and birth complications have significant but modest effect, in increasing the later risk of schizophrenia. Exposure to antepartum haemorrhage, diabetes, rhesus incompatibility, pre-eclampsia, low birth weight, congenital malformations, reduced head circumference, uterine atony, asphyxia and emergency caesarean section are some of the other risk factors (Cannon M, et al. 2002).

Advanced paternal age with increased risk for schizophrenia, have been repeatedly shown in people with no family history of the disorder. The possibility is of de-novo mutation in paternal sperm with ageing, in addition to exposure to micro-nutritional deficiencies such as folate (El-Saadi O, et al. 2004).

Cannabis usage as a risk factor is addressed in another chapter.

Etiology

The heritability of psychosis is estimated at approximately 40%; thus, environmental factors, moreover gene-environment interaction, plays a significant role in the susceptibility for, and progression, of a psychotic illness (Van Os J, et al. 2010). The association between childhood adversity, trauma and psychosis is now well accepted, associated with higher level of positive psychotic symptoms. Australian women are likely to be 3 times more, sexually abused than men, posing it as a risk factor.

The identification of trauma in psychotic population should be included, as part of routine clinical assessment, and in the development of appropriate mental health treatment plans.

However the etiology remains elusive, with predominant hypothesis of a neurodevelopmental disorder, and strong genetic predisposition, interacting with environmental risk factors, altering shape and size of developing neural structure. It is likely that multiple genetic factors that influence brain development, glial cell structure and function, and wide range of other neurochemicals, neuro-hormonal, circadian and neuro-immunological factors: are all relevant. Many of the genetic risks, appear to be shared with other major psychiatric disorders, like bipolar disorder and early childhood brain development disorders, such as autism (Hickie IB, et al. 2009).

First-episode schizophrenia patients, and their unaffected siblings might share regional white matter deficit in frontal and temporal lobes. White matter abnormalities are likely to cause disintegration of neural activity, and communications, and thereby cognitive dysfunction.

Males are more likely to develop schizophrenia than females, suggesting the moderating effect of oestrogen. Clinical evidence, epidemiological findings and animal studies have pointed towards the neuro-protective role of oestrogen. It is certainly a useful concept, worth exploring the enigma of schizophrenia. Decline in oestrogen levels, is associated with later onset of schizophrenia, exacerbation of psychosis, poor outcome and lower antipsychotic response.

Other emerging theories are; of autoimmune disorder and neuromuscular synapse formation, which is either deficient during childhood or excessively pruned during adolescence.

I never felt comfortable with the theory of "high expressed emotion" which was prevalent during my training period of 1970s. Patients' families were excluded from any management plan, in the name of creating negative home environment and causing the illness. This, I believed: was anti therapeutic. Thankfully it has been replaced by family's inclusion, and also recognised for the significant contribution they make, in recovery and care. In a Cochrane analysis, psycho education program among caregivers, showed the potential for higher level of compliance, lower rate of relapse and improved psychopathological status (Pekala, E et al.2002).

Pathophysiology

Schizophrenia has been conceptualised as the disorder of disrupted structural brain connectivity, accompanied by a functional miscommunication between different brain areas. These structural brain abnormalities are thought, to stem from early developmental processes, linked to genetic, prenatal and environmental factors; before the full blown symptoms, progressing over time, after illness onset, and as psychosis develop: specially in the grey matter areas (Kochunov P, et al. 2014).

To explain the breakdown of neural machinery, Davies et al proposed the theory of neuro-progression, that the clinical syndrome of schizophrenia, arises in susceptible people via accumulation of multiple negative 'events' starting in utero and in perinatal period. It involves complex epigenetic changes, which together, lead to the increased expression of abnormal inflammatory markers, such as tryptophan, catabolites, and reactive oxygen species: damaging to the developing brain. The toxic combination of these markers impacted by other negative 'events' like underperforming NMDA receptors and/

or methylation abnormalities cause the growth and development of abnormal neuronal circuit, seen in schizophrenia.

The later negative 'events' like cannabis or stimulant use, social adversity such as bullying, migration, family stress, childhood trauma, social isolation and affective changes play important role.

The brain changes, in the first year of illness appear to be especially prominent as compared in the later stages. Neurobiology of mental illness is highly dynamic, depending on the stage of the illness, and effectiveness of interventions. There are several brain regions, which show abnormality from the outset, and gradually progress. Ventricular enlargement, grey matter decline, and hippocampal volume reduction, present in first episode psychosis, are consistently observed in the chronic stage, suggesting its potential as a biological risk marker. Longitudinal early psychosis literature suggests, that the brain continues to develop abnormally, for at least several years, following initial onset of illness; giving it tacit support for being a progressive illness (Andreasen NC, et al. 2011).

It is postulated that early stages of schizophrenia, psychotic depression, and bipolar disorder, present with a generic phenotype, dominated by nonspecific features like depression, odd thoughts, irritability, inattention, cognitive impairment, circadian rhythm disturbance, social withdrawal, anxiety and periodic agitation. I guess it is similar to the early concepts of diagnosing illnesses, when Kraepelin separated manic-depressive insanity from dementia praecox. It is best described as the trunk and branch model, which proposes that this undifferentiated phenotype is the consequence of one or more pathophysiological mechanisms acting during the post-pubertal phase of development. During this key phase of life, other biological changes are also taking place, like central corticotrophin releasing factor resistance, disturbed circadian function, abnormal pattern of synaptic pruning, dys-regulated central neuro immune function and reduced production of brain derived neuro trophic factor (BDNF) (Banati R, et al 2009).

The onset period of the illness is correlated with the critical late phase of synaptic pruning in the prefrontal lobe. Synapse (the brain communicator) density reaches its peak just before adolescence then decreases by at least 30% during adolescent years and remains constant thereafter till after 70 years of age. People with schizophrenia have excessive regression of synapses (of about 60%) in the dorsolateral prefrontal cortex.

However the question still remains unresolved; if many synapses fail to form during childhood or there is excessive pruning, during adolescence (Bennett MR. 2008)?

The trunk and branch concept is useful, in understanding the progress of pathophysiological changes of psychiatric illnesses, and emergence of more distinct and discerning clinical features. Genetic predisposition, intrauterine infection, early childhood abuse and infections or brain trauma, as well as alcohol or substance misuse, or psychosocial trauma may delineate the course of the branches of the trunk.

The innate immune system of brain is Microglia. The biological stress of psychotic illness for prolonged period that leads to decline in general health, also maintains microglia in persistently reactive state, a feature of schizophrenia.

Hyper-prolactinaemia is commonly observed in people with psychotic disorders as well as the side effect of neuroleptic medication, due to D2 receptor blockade by antipsychotic drugs. It may also exist in drug naïve patients with first episode psychosis. High levels have been associated with sexual dysfunction, galactorrhoea, amenorrhoea, osteoporosis and cognitive impairment; more in men than women.

There have been several reports linking delusion of pregnancy with antipsychotic induced hyper-prolactinaemia (Hu LY 2015). The patient, as the delusional belief, can misinterpret both amenorrhoea and abdominal distension, caused by elevated prolactin level.

Any research in schizophrenia is challenging, due to effects of antipsychotic medication and factors secondary to the illness, like substance abuse or life style issues of reduced physical activities and diminished cognitive challenges.

Prodrome

Schizophrenia is usually preceded by sustained and prolonged period of emotional and behavioural changes, which may include social cognition: mental operations underlying social interactions. The symptoms may vary in intensity and clarity and may be overlooked. This may lead to gradual or sudden, sub threshold or fluctuating emergence of more diagnostic symptoms of delusions or hallucinations. It needs special attention to assess these symptoms, as preventive measures, in addition to lifestyle factors, like inactivity, smoking and unhealthy dietary choices, rendering them more prone to develop the illness.

Early psychosis intervention remains controversial till date, between early diagnosis and assertive treatment; to delayed diagnosis and delayed treatment, for the reasons of its emotional impact, and adverse reactions of the antipsychotic drugs. Schizophrenia goes from being relatively treatment responsive disorder at the first presentation to treatment resistant in multi-episode patients (Catts SV et al 2016).

Prospective memory is impaired in patients with schizophrenia, which is inability to remember to carry out an intended action in the future. Cue identification (going to shop) and intention retrieval (to buy milk) are the components of prospective memory. It has been suggested that prospective memory deficit in schizophrenia is a primary deficit, rather than secondary consequence of cognitive impairment. There is promising work being done, using cue identification and, intention retrieval as a potential biomarker for early detection, treatment and prognosis of schizophrenia (Chengfeng Ji, et al 2017).

Impairments of neurocognitive functions; are considered as core features of, schizophrenia, since patients show substantial decline at the onset of the disease and impairment persists even after remission of psychotic symptoms. Children who later develop schizophrenia lag behind developmentally in multiple neurocognitive domains with delayed premorbid development. Ultra high-risk individuals would show generalised neurocognitive impairment as prodromal sign that falls between patients with first episode schizophrenia and healthy controls (Bang M, et al 2015).

Impressive work is done in Australia, highlighting preclinical and prodromal symptoms heralding the possibility of a disordered mind, like impaired social functioning in the areas of communication, employment and general competence. There is a significant relationship between clinical symptoms, neurocognitive and social functioning. If identified earlier it may be amenable to prevention strategies, improving final outcome and transition to psychosis (McGorry, et al).

Early detection and reducing the duration of untreated psychosis, has long term effect, on transition into a full blown illness, remission, relapse prevention, hospitalisations, treatment engagement and recovery. However, no one type of intervention seems to be, superior to any other, in preventing the transition to psychosis.

There is some evidence of positive effect of cognitive behavioural therapy on distress associated with psychotic experiences.

The available literature on prevention strategies still remains divided as the following studies.

1. Antipsychotic administration to high-risk patients is potentially harmful with no preventive benefit, it may provide symptomatic benefit without functional outcome': from a large-scale longitudinal study (Zhang TH, et al. 2020).

   It is possible to reduce the risk of developing psychotic disorder in those with high risk for up to 4 years, early intervention improves outcome across the early years of illness (Fusar-Poli P, et al. 2017).

2. "There are major risks in using antipsychotic medications, for its adverse effect on weight gain, metabolic syndrome and diabetes. Recent evidence is that it may be associated with brain atrophy, and these medications may induce psychiatric symptoms in people, who are not psychotic. There are major risks in using antipsychotic medication for early intervention of psychosis, which researchers must take into account and inform participants about" (Jorm A F. 2012).

Diagnosis

> *'It is more important to know the patient who has the disease than the disease the patient has'.*
>
> Hippocrates 480 BC

There have been advances in refining the diagnosis, acknowledging multiple domains impacting on the disease process and possible preventions.

Apart from first rank symptoms, depression is not uncommon in schizophrenia, which can be misinterpreted, for negative symptoms like apathy, lack of motivation and withdrawal. Patient may gain insight upon recovery, precipitating reactive depression. Post psychotic depression may also result from loss of psychotic grandiosity, delusions and hallucination, which may have provided the apparent purpose and occupation during the illness. The treatment may also contribute to depression, such as dopamine blockade, by antipsychotic medication and extra pyramidal symptoms, mimicking depression.

History taking, mental state, and neurological examination, have remained the mainstay of any psychiatric diagnosis including schizophrenia, above any neuroimaging investigation till now.

Schizophrenia and violence

Mental illness does not necessarily cause offending, but it may compromise well being, precluding optimal functioning and problem solving skills, inducing susceptibility to other risk factors and rendering interventions difficult.

However people affected with schizophrenia spectrum disorders are, at the higher risk of offending. Unfortunately this has been the general public perception without considering the factors, which provokes the antisocial behaviour of a person, with schizophrenia. Male gender, past history of violence, comorbid substance abuse, lower educational attainment and unemployment are, more prevalent in the violent subgroup in addition to, history of family conflicts necessitating police intervention, before the diagnosis of schizophrenia. Emerging evidence indicates that first episode psychosis may represent a particularly high-risk period for the occurrence of violence

Co-morbidity, in the form of personality disorders and/or substance use disorder is frequent. These findings suggest that lower level of social functioning, is possibly related to higher degree of antisocial traits. Following the diagnosis of schizophrenia, the increased risk for violence can be assumed by, higher numbers and longer duration of inpatient care, higher rate of non-compliance and severe positive symptoms.

Assessment of a person with schizophrenia should include the potential for violence even if it is to minimal level (Large MM, et al 2011).

Treatment

As with any illness, treatment remains the ultimate and most significant goal. For schizophrenia, it is even more vital, due to its profound impact, not only, on the patient but everyone connected to them. The human cost of the illness, is totally encompassing. The financial cost which can be measured, and is necessary for the health budget planning, is anywhere between $4000 and $12,000, depending on inpatient, outpatient, relapse and rehospitalisation, over a period of 12 months for each patient (Carl VJ, et al. 2003).

The treatment of Schizophrenia remains just as challenging. Over the past 30 years, several atypical antipsychotic drugs were introduced, hoping to safely replace the older drugs. Unfortunately NIMH sponsored trial in US, CATIE (clinical antipsychotic trial of interventional effectiveness) was unconvincing, of the superiority of second generation anti psychotics, against the first generation, apart from modest benefits, and variable adherence. A decade later, the largest meta-analysis of cohort study was published, refuting the claim and asserting that these medications, slowed or reversed the accelerated rate of grey matter volume loss, observed in first episode schizophrenia patients (Vita A, et al. 2015). This interpretation is consistent with evidence of neurotropic actions of these drugs.

The Australian National Survey of People living with Psychosis, carried out 10 years apart (1998-2010), concluded that there were no measurable improvements, in major indicators of disability. Additionally there was almost doubling of rates of lifetime drug and alcohol abuse, while government expenditure on public mental health services, more than doubled over the same period.

Approximately 20-30% of people with schizophrenia do not respond to treatment (Agid, O, et al.2011).

Presence of negative symptoms and cognitive impairment, are the most resistant aspect of the illness, most vital for recovery, and most challenging, to treat.

Once the diagnosis of schizophrenia is established, and the treatment commenced, maintenance antipsychotic medication should be, continued indefinitely, to prevent relapses. Psychotic relapses contribute substantially, to poor long-term outcome. Long acting injectable antipsychotic medications are more effective in preventing relapses (Catts S V, 2016).

For safe administration of antipsychotic drugs regular monitoring of a range of cardio-metabolic parameters is recommended which should include prolactin levels, renal and liver functions, bone indices and creatine kinase.

Concurrent use of 2 or more antipsychotic drugs is polypharmacy which remains controversial. It increases adverse effects, lowers patient compliance and not recommended by treatment guidelines (Geoff DC et-al 2011).

One of the most concerning side effects of antipsychotic medication is tardive dyskinesia, as it can cause permanent impairment, with little recourse. Although it is often thought of being rare with 2nd generation antipsychotics, the literature is divided over its frequency.

There is more evidence-based support for clozapine mono-therapy. Relapse prevention remains the most modifiable risk factor, for emergent treatment resistance.

Clozapine: was reintroduced for the treatment of resistant patients, in 1993 though not without its serious adverse reactions, and mandatory regular monitoring.

Most of the psychotropic drugs, including antidepressants and antipsychotics, specially, clozapine, need to be assessed for the balance of benefit and harm. Sudden cardiac death has been reported with QT-prolongation: potential risk of torsades-de-pointes, which, indicates for regular ECGs, at least for the inpatients. Cardio-metabolic side effects of clozapine are well recognised, and mostly included in the treatment plan.

Cardiomyopathy (echocardiographic evidence) which can occur, months or years after commencing clozapine, and myocarditis (rise in C-reactive protein) within a few months, are the potential severe adverse reactions, related to clozapine use.

Rates of clozapine-induced myocarditis appear to be higher in Australia, than other countries (Lambert T 2010). The veracity of the diagnosis of clozapine-induced myocarditis may be suboptimal, therefore it should be confirmed and consulted, before the decision to cease. Clozapine should be justifiably rechallenged as evidenced by recently published reports, though under strict and rigorous monitoring protocol.

For the benefit of continuing clozapine, there should be regular monitoring of emerging cardiac pathology.

Photosensitivity reactions in the form of hyperpigmentation, is a known side effect of the First-generation antipsychotics and antidepressant medications. It is associated with long-term use and is generally irreversible (Mendhkar ND. 2009).

Another serious side effect is, severe constipation, which may result in bowel obstruction, due to slow gastrointestinal transit, as the result of its significant anticholinergic effect and serotonin receptor antagonism (Every-Palmer S, et al.2017). It can cause mucosal ischemia and necrosis leading to gastrointestinal perforation and toxic megacolon. This is a significant and potentially fatal adverse effect, which should be mitigated with laxatives. Gastric reflux secondary to gastric hypo-motility is a, common complaint. There have been, several reported deaths in Australia, associated with clozapine induced gastric hypo-motility.

Nocturnal enuresis, priapism and seizure are less common side effects. Clozapine-induced neutropenia and agranulocytosis, are the major concerns in prescribing this drug, which requires its mandatory regular monitoring at least in Australia. Clozapine being the most effective treatment for treatment resistant schizophrenia, its apparent adverse effects should be well explored, before the decision to cease. There is reported benign ethnic neutropenia, as the common cause of chronic neutropenia in many ethnic communities, like African and people from Middle Eastern descent. It does not increase the risk of agranulocytosis and has led to threshold modification in monitoring the guidelines in US, UK and Ireland (Bray A 2008).

One potentially lethal side effect is, neuroleptic malignant syndrome (NMS) characterised by, muscle rigidity, hyperthermia, autonomic instability, leucocytosis, mental state changes, and evidence of muscle injury (elevated creatinine kinase). It is a medical emergency (Strawn JR, et al. 2007). Atypical NMS, a variant of NMS, with variation in abnormal values, as well as other symptoms of sudden confusion, incontinence, and unsteady gait can make the diagnosis difficult.

Reduction in dopaminergic activity in the brain, probably by D2 receptor blockade in the striatum and hypothalamus, is considered a potential cause of NMS (Gillman PK. 2010).

Troublesome hypotension can appear, as late as 6 months into the treatment, and may be severe enough to warrant clozapine suspension. Aripiprazole with its unique pharmacological profile of, high affinity partial agonist at dopaminergic D2 and D3 receptors, and serotonergic 5–HT1A receptors, as well as antagonism at 5-HT2A and 5-HT2C, similar to the receptor profile of N-desmethyl-clozapine, can be a successful switch from Clozapine (Burris KD, et al. 2002).

Increased odds of developing venous thromboembolism and pulmonary embolism have been reported with other antipsychotic drugs as well as clozapine. In patients treated with clozapine, the modifiable risks of pulmonary-embolism must be considered important.

Hyper-salivation is a common side effect, which can be associated with aspiration pneumonia. Atropine 1% eye drops applied sublingually has been found effective in controlling this embarrassing symptom.

One has to be mindful that clozapine levels can markedly increase following abrupt smoking cessation leading to dose dependent side effects. Some psychotropic medications like SSRI and haloperidol can change plasma clozapine levels to toxicity by inhibiting CYP2D6. Additionally, caffeine consumption, stress, hypo-albuminaemia, renal and hepatic failure as well as infections; have potential to increase clozapine level.

There are significant individual and ethnic differences in clozapine absorption and metabolism. The levels are generally higher in female than males.

Plasma clozapine levels between 350 to 400 microgram/ml, were significantly associated with improved clinical response rate, for patients with schizophrenia (Lopez LV, et al 2013).

There is also evidence that levels above 600 micrograms/ml, can increase risk of seizures, and so do the co-prescription of certain SSRI like fluvoxamine.

Although clozapine is the most effective drug for refractory schizophrenia, 40% of patients do not meet the response criteria. Therefore augmentation strategies must be the next option. Having optimised the clozapine dosage, aripiprazole, fluoxetine and along with promising result of ECT can be considered (Tully J, et al. 2016).

However use of sodium valproate in women of childbearing age must be with extreme caution due to its teratogenic potential.

The potential role of neuroimaging and biomarker in guiding the treatment selection will open the doors, not only for medication but also predicting response to psychological and cognitive therapies. For example reduced plasma level of BDNF may indicate the need to use medications and greater cortical reserve may predict response to CBT

Evidence suggests that both cognitive behavioral therapy for psychosis and cognitive remediation are helpful for person with schizophrenia.

Although it may not directly address the psychopathology but improves thinking, concentration and learning which can make substantial gain.

The Schizophrenia Research Institute estimates that schizophrenia will cost Australia AUD 2.6 billions per annum unless treatments are optimised. Combining psychosocial treatments in comprehensive management plan is overdue. With sufficient evidence that CBT and cognitive remediation play a significant role in recovery, these treatment modalities need further exploration and enhancement.

Pregnancy and schizophrenia

The prevalence of mental disorders in pregnant women is high. Perinatal-mental health therefore must begin, from preconception planning through to pregnancy, until 3 years post-partum, which is vital.

Prevention begins from the time a fetus is conceived when neurological development is most vulnerable. Understanding the role of fetal programming in schizophrenia is likely to be central, to the goal of prevention (Debnath M, et al 2014).

The risks for women with schizophrenia start, with unplanned pregnancy, suboptimal antenatal nutrition and care, higher rate of maternal obesity and substance abuse.

Unfortunately the studies on this group of patients are confounded by, their life-style issues, like alcohol and substance abuse, noncompliance, smoking, use of multiple psychotropic drugs and obesity. Moreover, schizophrenia and bipolar disorders are associated with, an increased risk of adverse birth outcome regardless of treatment (Boden R, et al 2012b).

Psychotic episode during pregnancy doubles the rate of adverse pregnancy outcomes (Nilsson E, et al 2008).

Although there is limited evidence of birth defects or complications, women on long term and high dosage of anti psychotic medication are likely to have preterm birth, neonatal abstinence syndrome as well as gestational diabetes and hypertension. Therefore it is prudent to be mindful of the risks and benefits of prescribing antipsychotic medications, which is also increasingly being used off label.

Parenting in Schizophrenia

Importance of good parenting cannot be underestimated as it shapes child's growth and development across all spheres and also fosters psychological development of the parent.

Comprehensive integrated care of pregnant women with schizophrenia, should be high priority for perinatal mental health, and maternity services. Parenting capacity, transition to motherhood, and maternal bonding, must be the key parts of perinatal and postnatal care.

Australian and international data suggests that around 50% women with schizophrenia, will have involvement with child protection services, and about 40% of their children will be placed, in residential care at sometime during their childhood (Ranning A, et al. 2015).

Separation and loss suffered by the parent, and the child must be acknowledged.

Majority of the parents with psychosis, living with their dependent children, were found to function well with regards to quality of care, according to the Second Australian National Survey of Psychosis. Nevertheless there is significant minority of parents with obvious and severe impairment in their ability, to care for their children even after, clinical recovery. In some studies mothers with schizophrenia were found to be remote, silent, self-absorbed, verbally and behaviorally intrusive, flaccid, insensitive and unresponsive, with fewer mutually satisfying interactions (Wan MW, et al 2007) resulting in disrupted bonding.

Collaboration between obstetrics and mental health services remains, an important part of care during and after pregnancy.

Discussing with women of childbearing age, about their plan for pregnancy needs to include information, about its potential risks to the mother and the child.

Focus on parenting for women with schizophrenia should be considered, central to a recovery paradigm. Understanding and modifying risk factors in the pathways, from one to next generation, is the outset of best preventative measure.

Novel Therapeutic Possibilities

Recognition of neuro-protective agents, promoting neurogenesis and maintaining synaptic plasticity in the brain, has opened a new corridor of possibilities, for treating schizophrenia, both in early and late stages.

Essential fatty acids, by reducing oxidative stress, are safe and well tolerated excellent agents, for trial in treating mental illnesses (Ross BM, et al. 2007).

Feeding the brain with essential fatty acids, is the subject of several promising clinical trials, on the hypothesis that omega-3 polyunsaturated fatty acids (PUFAs) play an important role, in preventing the conversion of prodromal stage to full blown psychosis. There are suggestions of using PUFAs, in prodromal stage.

Lithium with its potent neuro protective property has been shown, to be effective in the treatment of degenerative neurological disorders, associated with increase in grey matter. There are some reported positive outcomes of symptomatic response of Lithium, in psychotic symptoms.

Dysregulation of HPA (hypothalamic pituitary adrenal) axis occurs in response to stress and trauma, with changes in the volume of key brain structures, specially, pituitary and hippocampus. There are possible interventions currently on trial, to moderate the impact of stress and trauma.

N–acetyl cysteine, a neuro protective has been found useful in reducing oxidative stress. It may be useful adjunct to standard treatment, for the improvement of negative and total schizophrenia symptoms, as well as cognitive domain of working memory.

Psychotropic medication may recruit compensatory brain processes that oppose, the initial positive effect of the drug. Therefore prolonged use of medication may worsen at least in some cases, patient's long-term clinical and functional outcome (Mulder R, et al 2017). So there is a strong message that pharmacotherapy may not provide, all our answers to treat mental illnesses.

In Australia, people with Schizophrenia, suffer the most stress from poor finances, social isolation, loneliness and unemployment, impacting on their physical and mental health, which must be addressed for any therapeutic benefit.

With the complexity of illness, the treatment is multilevel, including neurological, cognitive and social functioning. Social functioning deficit is a trait and state marker of risk for serious mental disorders. Access to meaningful work has been recognised as a significant factor in the recovery of mental illnesses: unfortunately it has never been developed to its full potential. The unemployment rate amongst mentally ill patients is 75 to 80 %, against the general population average of 5%. The usual options of sheltered workshops, voluntary work, like car wash, mowing, catering, and similar jobs are not generously available, and may not maximise their vocational potential.

Recreational and occupational activities though acknowledged; not universally implemented as part of recovery.

Social skills training during remission period is vital, to maximise the enduring and satisfactory personal relationships, which must be a serious consideration in recovery.

The concept of comprehensive care plan, to return the patient to their maximal/optimal premorbid function, is neither new nor limited to psychiatry though it is still staggering, to find its place in everyday life of a psychiatric patient.

It was interesting to note from the annals of history, that Dr Attfield the Surgeon Superintendent of Fremantle Asylum advocated self discipline, cleanliness, recreation and abolition of mechanical restraints in his treatment of mentally ill. He provided all possible amusements and indulgence in the form of books, cricket, draughts and several ball games in the Warehouse asylum of Western Australia in 1857. (Ellis AS 19084).

Recovery

The definition of recovery has changed, with the widening affluence, mechanisation and technology. Symptom relief is not the only goal of the mentally ill person: who is expected to return to as much a functional life as possible which includes, self-acceptance, the capacity to see and accept one's strength and weaknesses, having goals and objectives, that gives life, meaning and directions, even with limitations caused by illness. It must complement personal growth realising talents and potential; positive relations with others with close and valued connections; environmental mastery, and being able to manage the demands of everyday life and autonomy.

Recovery is deeply personal unique process of changing one's attitude, values, feelings, goals, skills and roles. It involves development of new meaning and purpose in life as one grows beyond the catastrophic effects of mental illness (Slade 2009).

The role of occupational therapist in recovery is important to help patients become more productive. Employment opportunities must be explored and developed to help people re-enter the challenging workforce for productive and vocational participation in the ongoing journey of recovery (Harvey et al 2013).

Money, social engagement and employment are the most important challenges for people with psychotic illness, as well as good physical and mental health. With the complexity of the illness and limited response to medication, the role of evidence-based psychosocial therapy must be, vital part of the management plan.

A structure, which enables the consumer to participate actively, in their assessment, is a fundamental first step, towards recovery-oriented practice. Active participation by the consumer, in their own assessment, and treatment planning, facilitates self-direction and empowerment: repeatedly described as core recovery process (Bird V, et al. 2014).

Recovery Assessment Scale-Domains and Stages (RAS-DS) is an effective and efficient instrument that generates, valid and reliable scores reflecting mental health recovery It promotes understanding and partnership between the consumer and the staff, as a basis of collaborative intervention planning.

Cognitive remediation and cognitive enhancement, recognises more malleable nature of cognitive difficulties, in everyday life of a psychiatric patient.

Club House/ Fountain House was established in 1948, by the ex patients of New York psychiatric hospital, for developing a potentially robust and comprehensive program for not only symptom removal, but returning the patients to maximum functionality. The scheme was half-heartedly adapted in Australia, which unfortunately never flourished.

Housing is central to building a future. There is growing body of evidence that housing plays important role in recovery. It is even more critical for people with Schizophrenia. The positive gains of inpatient treatment must be complemented by suitable and secure housing, independence, relationships, activities and general quality of life.

Due to nature of psychiatry, the therapeutic relationship is far more personal both for doctor and the patient, an important consideration in recovery.

So there is no surprise, that in addition to symptoms of the disorder, there are reactionary emotional overload, of fear, anxiety, perplexity and demoralisation, no less in the patients with schizophrenia, than any other illness. Exploring patients inner world generate countertransference in the doctor, wanting to take full responsibility for healing, with overdeveloped sense of professional and personal responsibility, for the welfare of their patients. How many of us can deny this paternalistic feeling?

Remission: Inevitability of poor outcome for patients with schizophrenia has been successfully challenged with advancing research (De Hert M, et al. 2007).

In 2005, the Remission in Schizophrenia Working Group (RSWG) conceptualized remission criteria, for schizophrenia. It was defined by both a severity and a time criterion. Remission is achieved when the core symptoms like positive, negative and disorganisation do not exceed a score of mild, for at least 6 months (Andreasen NC et al. 2005). Superior premorbid functioning, younger age, shorter illness, social cognition, less severe symptoms and better medication adherence, favour symptomatic improvement and remission. RSWG also emphasized that for recovery, the individual must have, subjective appraisal of satisfaction with life and daily activities, suitable functioning in everyday life, as well as adaptation to live beyond the absence of, psychopathology.

We often forget the role of carers, in the care of our severely disabled patients. Although carers and families of people with mental illness are; crucial part of health and community support system, their experiences are rarely explored systematically

Research has consistently found that relatives who care for the mentally ill person have increased risk of post-traumatic stress disorder. The carers are subjected to constraints on their work, finance, social and leisure activities, marital relationships and intimacy together with detrimental effect, on their mental and emotional wellbeing. Adverse interactions between people with mental disorder and their intimate partner or other family members, predicts poor outcome, in contrast to supportive family environment, which has better outcome (Review 2003-2008).

The legitimate role of carers and families within our health-care system requires, their formal recognition and promotion. Beyond Blue has, national association, Blue-Voices promoting interests of people with depression and their carers as well as families.

Mental health legislation and policy formation have highlighted: family involvement as the key issue, in the current care environment for a person suffering from severe mental illness. Yet in spite of theses legal and policy initiatives, the involvement of family carers is far from satisfactory.

Barriers to involvement of family and carers must be overcome, if better outcome for their mentally ill relatives is to be achieved.

RANZCP Community Collaboration Committee is a joint Tasman partnership of consumers, carers, RANZCP Fellows and trainees. Established in 1996, it advocates for better participatory, patient centered, mental health care. It acts as a conduit between the needs of community and psychiatry.

Despite the progress, neuroscience has made in the field of schizophrenia, there is a wide gap, between what is possible and what is available, both nationally and internationally (Catts S V et al 2016).

In two last major national surveys, the conclusion was; that health and social status of people with schizophrenia has barely improved over the years, and it is far below what is possible.

Case Study

I met this attractive mother of 3 sons in her mid twenties. This was her first hospital admission after the birth of her youngest son. She grew up on a farm in a small country town, often cared by her grandmother, as her mother suffered from Schizophrenia and needed frequent and long hospitalisations in 1960s.

She was a bright affable and an emotionally sensitive girl. She completed her higher school certificate and moved to Sydney for city life. She worked, lived independently, and met her future husband with no sign of, prodromal symptom, indicative of, genetic loading. The diagnosis of post partum psychosis after the delivery of her third child, decompensated her underlying fear, she always had, of going the path of her mother.

Her discharge home was followed by a decade of turbulence when her family life fell apart, she started to drink, involving in inappropriate relationships with other hospital patients and requiring increasing dosages of antipsychotic medications along with the adverse drug effects, and recurring hospitalisations with florid psychosis. Her husband a conscientious and a supportive man, could no longer care for the family with the disruptions caused by his wife's illness, so he left the family home and their children.

After a few more relapses the patient started to stabilise, became cooperative and compliant when we engaged in regular therapy sessions. She gradually reconnected with her children to the extent of providing care for her grandchildren on regular basis. She maintained cordial relationship with her now ex-husband who by then remarried, which she accepted without any malice. She started visiting her family on the farm and actively participated in family decisions.

Her only sister to whom she was emotionally close died tragically after a debilitating illness. Her ability to cope with the loss and keep the family together, was exemplary. I continued to see her regularly and together we made the decision to minimise her medication, planning to cease when she felt confident. Her appointment intervals gradually became longer as she gained control of her life, though I continued to receive warm and caring letters from her.

She taught me a lot about life, resilience, compromises and forgiveness, and most of all, the power of human relationships, which can melt many obstacles in life, including schizophrenia, though the lost years of life can never be returned.

After over 3 decades of seeing each other, sharing her inner-most thoughts and feelings, how can I not have the sense of responsibility, fondness and loyalty.

Comorbidity

Most psychiatric illnesses specially schizophrenia, have increased propensity for poor health like obesity and smoking and long term poorer outcome. It may be biological or due to lifestyle factors. Therefore screening for physical health must be essential part of initial assessment in schizophrenia.

Comorbidity in schizophrenia is a significant issue, for bio-psychosocial reasons, as well as inactive lifestyle, smoking and low dietary fibre intake. Mortality rate for people with schizophrenia is excessive and premature: cardiovascular diseases are the major cause of it. The significant risk factors for increased morbidity and mortality are, more prevalent in schizophrenia. The predictor of cardiovascular diseases, obesity, diabetes, dyslipidemia and smoking are far more common, than the general population. They also have more prevalent family history of cardio-vascular diseases and diabetes. Unfortunately most of the antipsychotic medications also have the potential to worsen these pre existing symptoms.

The high prevalence, of people with schizophrenia and alcohol/substance abuse comorbidity is complex, challenging and substantial. My experience with the patients presented to the Mental Health Review Tribunal for Community Treatment Orders was, that at least 80% had comorbid drug and alcohol issues, which unfortunately was not in the plan of the treatment.

The dilemma has been the lack of integrated health care of mentally ill patients. There is poor coordination between primary and secondary care. Psychiatrists focus on mental health issues, and non-psychiatrist doctors, are reticent to treat people with mental illnesses. These patients have more frequent contacts with their case managers who are either non-medical or of nursing background and with frequent changeovers, where the physical complaints are generally brushed off.

In late 2016 Australian Government announced funding, for patients with complex and severe mental illness, to receive integrated health care package delivered through primary health services. This was supported by RANZCP, highlighting the importance of communication, collaboration and partnership, between mental health professionals and the general practitioners, who are visited by mentally ill people, more often than they visit their psychiatrist.

The challenges on patient side may be, due to cognitive impairment or socially isolated life. They may find difficult to comprehend and follow the advice of health maintenance issues.

Vitamin D There is robust evidence indicating suboptimal vitamin D status, among 31% Australians (Daly RM, et al.2012).

It is much worse in people with physical or psychiatric illness due to reduced outdoor activities. People with psychotic disorders are at the risk of developing cardio-metabolic disease, which is further accentuated by low vitamin D, as well as compounded by the adverse effects of neuroleptics, like raised prolactin levels.

There is also evidence that neonatal vitamin D deficiency is associated with, increased risk of schizophrenia.

Routine monitoring of vitamin D as well as improving physical health status must be part of comprehensive management plan.

Obstructive sleep apnoea: (OSA) Characterised by repeated occlusions to the upper-airway, during periods of nocturnal sleep, resulting in snoring, nocturnal hypoxemia, fragmented sleep, and daytime symptoms like irritability, reduced affect, and reduced quality of life (Engleman H, et al. 2004). There is significant comorbidity of depression and insomnia possibly with bidirectional relationship, both for symptoms and recovery.

OSA is more than 3 times commoner in schizophrenia (Miles H, et al.2016). These patients are often fatigued, despite their seemingly long hours of sleep, which has poor quality and they complain of restless legs. These symptoms need investigations for possible treatable cause.

OSA contributes to cardio-metabolic risks. Untreated OSA increases, oxidative stress and sympathetic activation, which exacerbate hypertension, insulin resistance, heart-failure and atrial fibrillation.

There is documented improvement in insomnia, daytime drowsiness and depressive symptoms following the application of Continuous Positive Air Pressure (CPAP) therapy. Treatment of underlying depression has been shown to improve OSA symptom outcome, with adherence to CPAP.

According to RANZCP Clinical Practice Guidelines for Schizophrenia, it is imperative to assess OSA, by questioning about daytime somnolence, snoring and breathing pauses. By treating OSA and reducing somnolence, physical quality of life, is likely to improve.

Blood-borne virus: Patients with severe mental illness have several times higher prevalence of blood born virus infection. Most common are hepatitis C and B viruses as well as HIV. It is even higher in needle syringe exchangers and the prison population.

Psychosis or Schizophrenia like symptoms can arise from legal or illegal drugs as well. Both SSRI and SNRI have been reported to cause symptoms of delusions, ideas of references, agitation without any cognitive impairment

Folie a deux

This shared psychotic disorder has total of 18 names including double insanity, psychosis of association and induced delusional disorder etc. Although it has been known for 150 years, remains an elusive entity (Mergui J 2010). It is defined by presence of similar psychotic symptoms in 2 or more individuals living together, so the delusion of primary patient is adopted by the partner in an over dependent relationship.

Case Study

A 47 years old single woman on disability pension was referred to see me for her uncooperative, threatening behaviour with paranoid thoughts, about her sister who lived next door. She was living with her 82 years old father since her mother died nearly 10 years ago. Although she was high functioning, managed her home well and was talented in needlework, remained socially isolated. She was generally distrustful and occasionally made claims of suspicion against other people, including her sister confirming her paranoid delusions. On the day of her referral she went to the police station with her father, and both claimed that, their home was, infested by their neighbour, demanding that the police take action. Although she always harboured unusual thoughts and persecutory delusions, her father did not in the past. He was a hard working physically and mentally healthy man till his wife's death. He worked as a jeweler, before emigrating, from Europe. The patient's domineering and aggressive persona possibly kept her father under control, and he gradually started to share her delusional thinking to the extent of falsely accusing his older daughter and her family living next door. Whenever I challenged her delusional beliefs, her father confirmed it and supported her. Neither of them had any insight and defied my strong recommendation to take medication. They alienated most of their social network, and lived a stressful life, believing to be the victims. I was relieved to learn that following an aggressive episode on the street, both were hospitalized against their will.

Charles Bonnet Syndrome

This is a poorly understood disease, with optical illusions marked by distortion of shape, colour, motion and size. Unlike hallucinations, it has perceptual distortion of actual stimuli, like stationary object moving and straight lines may look wavy. Symptoms usually occur at night. Emergence of Lilliputian visual hallucinations, though the patient has insight, are distressing and puzzling to the person. Neither it is related to psychosis, nor has potential for dementia. There is underlying visual pathology, like macular degeneration, hemianopia, post eye surgery and pituitary-tumour, which needs to be addressed, to resolve the symptoms. Sometimes it is also referred as Alice in Wonderland Syndrome.

Case Study

A 76 years old lady was referred to see me by an ophthalmologist as an interesting case of vivid hallucinations, and patient's anxiety about possible mental illness. Apart from developing diminishing vision, she was in good health, living independently, occasionally taking care of her grandchildren and with reasonably active social life, interests and hobbies. There was no family history of any mental health issue.

She complained of vividly seeing children's birthday party in her backyard. Although she did not believe that the event was real, was extremely distressed by the vision from which she could not distract. I excluded other reasons for visual hallucination, like early dementia, stroke, Parkinson's disease, drug misuse and hormone replacement therapy, before reassuring her that she was not mentally ill.

I offered to prescribe anti anxiety or low dose antipsychotic, but more than that I reassured her to return to her referring specialist for more investigations. As there was no specific treatment, she was prepared to watch and wait.

Creutzfeldt-Jacob Disease (CJD)

Although it is a progressive neurodegenerative illness, in some cases psychiatric symptoms may be more prominent at the outset and can be misdiagnosed as schizophrenia. Impaired thinking possibly due to early dementia, personality changes, apathy mistaken for depression, can worsen as the disease progresses. It can be challenging for both psychiatrist as well as neurologist. A Heidenhain variant of CJD is characterized by complex visual hallucinations, affective symptoms as well as altered perception of colours and structure in the absence of typical cognitive and motor symptoms, in the early stage. It is easy to ignore or misdiagnose the neuropsychiatric symptoms. The presence of late onset unspecified visual symptoms in conjunction with affective or psychotic symptoms should include CJD in the differential diagnosis (Abudy A, et al 2014.).

Case Study

As part of deinstitutionalisation in mid seventies, we needed to review, all the long stay patients. An 82 years old man was transferred, from another hospital nearly 35 years earlier with no recorded family contact. His symptoms, on admission, and thereafter included, impaired memory, clumsiness, depressed mood, declining vision, unsteady gait and difficulty in communicating. Due to his occasional self-talk and delusional thinking which, may have been misinterpretation or fabrication, he was diagnosed and treated for schizophrenia. Magnetic

Resonance imaging and CSF, were not considered useful due to his length of hospitalisation and use of excessive psychotropic medications

A provisional diagnosis of CJD was made though could not be confirmed due to lack of relevant information. He died before his planned transfer to a nursing home for his long-term care. Autopsy was not considered, to confirm the diagnosis for various reasons.

CJD is a rare disease. During the recent times it first raised concerns in 1986 in UK, as a brain disorder linked to consuming meat from cattle, infected by bovine spongiform encephalopathy, informally known as mad cow disease.

The cause of CJD, are prion, a kind of protein essential for cell growth. However due to faulty folding /shaping, these prions become infectious, impeding the biological process, and creating spongy hole in the brain tissue.

Multiple Sclerosis: a disease characterised by focal areas of demyelination that can affect any part of the CNS resulting in varied signs and symptoms. There can be association between MS and psychosis. Apart from positive symptoms of hallucinations and delusions, fatigue and lethargy can be misinterpreted as negative symptoms.

References

Abudy A, Zohar et al 2014. The different faces of Creutzfeldt-Jacob Disease in psychiatry. General Hospital Psychiatry 36: 245-248.

Agid, O, Arenovich T et al. (2011) An algorithm based approach to first episode schizophrenia: Response rates over 3 prospective antipsychotic trials with a retrospective data analysis. Journal of Clinical Psychitry72: 1439-1444.

Andreasen NC, Carpenter WT, et al. 2005 Remission in schizophrenia: Proposed criteria and rationale for consensus. American Journal of Psychiatry 162: 441-449.

Andreasen NC, Nopoulos P, et al. 2011 Progressive brain change in schizophrenia; A prospective longitudinal study of first episode schizophrenia. Biological psychiatry. 70: 672-679.

Anthony, F Jorm. Ethics of giving antipsychotic medication to at-risk young people. Centre for Youth Mental Health ANZJP 2012 46 (9) 908-911.

Banati R, Hickie I. Therapeutic signposts: using biomarkers to guide better treatment of schizophrenia and other psychotic disorders. MJA Volume 190 Number 4 Feb 2009.

Bang M, Kyung RK, et al. Neurocognitive impairment in individuals at ultra high risk for psychosis: Who will really convert? ANZJP 2015 Vol 49 (5) 462-470.

Bennett MR. Dual constraint on synapse formation and regression in schizophrenia: neuregulin, neuroligin, dysbindin, DISCI, MuSK and agrin. ANZJP 2008; 42: 662-677.

Bird V, Leamy M, et al. 2014. Fit for purpose? Validation of a conceptual framework: for personal recovery with current mental health consumers. ANZJP 48: 644-653

Boden R, Lundgren M et al (2012b) risks of adverse pregnancy and birth outcomes in women treated or not treated with mood stabilisers for bipolar disorder: Population based cohort study. BMJ. 345: e7085

Bray A 2008. Ethnic neutropenia and clozapine, ANZJP 42: 342-345. Brown AS, Bottiglieri T, et al. Elevated prenatal homocysteine levels as a risk factor for schizophrenia. Arch Gen Psychiatry 2007; 64: 31-39.

Buka SL, Tsuang MT, et al. Maternal infections and subsequent psychosis among offspring. Arch GEN Psychiatry 2001; 58: 1032-10-37.

Burris KD, Molski TF, et al. 2002 Aripiprazole, a novel antipsychotic, is high affinity partial agonist at human dopamine D2 receptors. J Pharmacol Exp Ther 302:381-389

Cannon M, Jones PB et al. Obstetric complications and schizophrenia: historical and meta-analytic review. Amer J Psychiatry 2002; 159:1080-1092.

Cantor-Graae E, Selton JP. Schizophrenia and migration: a meta-analysis and review. Am J Psychiatry 2005; 162: 12-24.

Carl VJ, Neil AL, et al. Cost of schizophrenia and other psychoses in urban Australia: findings from low Prevalence Psychotic Disorders Study ANZ JP2003; 37: 31-40

Catts SV and O'Toole BI. The treatment of schizophrenia: Can we raise the standard of care? ANZJP 2016. Vol 50 (12) 1128-1138.

Chengfeng Ji, Dengtang L, et al. Impaired cue identification and intention retrieval underlie prospective memory deficits in patients with first episode schizophrenia. ANZJP 2017 Vol 51(3) 270-277.

Debnath M, Venkata-subramaniam G, et al. Foetal programming of schizophrenia: Select Mechanism, Neuroscience and Bio-behavioural Reviews, 2014. 49: 90-104.

Daly RM, Gagnon C, et-al.2012 Prevalence of vitamin D deficiency and its determinants in Australian adults aged 25 and older: A national, population based study. Clinical Endocrinology 77 26-35

De Hert M, van Winkle R, et al. 2007 Remission criteria for schizophrenia: Evaluation in large naturalistic cohort. Schizophrenia Research 92:68-73.

El-Saadi O, Pederson CB et al. Paternal and maternal age as risk factor for psychosis: findings from Denmark, Sweden and Australia. Schizophrenia Research 2004; 67:227-236.

Ellis AS; Eloquent Testimony: The Story of Mental Health Services in Western Australia 1830-1975, University of Western Australia Press, Nedlands, Western Australia1984.

Engleman H and Douglas n. 2004 Sleep.4: sleepiness, cognitive function and quality of life in obstructive sleep apnoea/hypopnoea syndrome Thorax 59: 618-622

Every-Palmer S, Newton-Howes G, et al.2017 Pharmacological treatment of anti-psychotic related constipation. Schizophrenia Bulletin 43:490-492.

Fusar-Poli P, McGory PD et al. 2017 Improving outcomes of first episode psychosis: An overview, World psychiatry 16: 251-265.

Geoff DC and Dixon L 2011 Antipsychotic poly-pharmacy: Are two ever better than one? American Journal of Psychiatry 168: 667-669.

Gillman PK. Neuroleptic malignant syndrome: mechanisms, interactions and causality. Mov Disord 2010; 25:1780-1790.

Harvey SB, Modini M, et al (2013) Severe mental illness and work: What can we do to maximise the employment opportunities for individuals with psychosis ANZJP Vol 47: 421-424.

Hickie IB, McGorry PD. Characterising novel pathways to schizophrenia. MJA. Volume 190 Number 4. Feb2009.

Hu LY, Lee YT et al. 2015 Using aripiprazole to treat new onset hyper prolactinimia related delusions of pregnancy. ANZJP 49; 946.

Jaaskelainen E, Juola P, et al. 2013. A systematic review and meta-analysis of recovery, in schizophrenia. Schizophrenia Bulletin. 39: 1296-1306.

Kochunov P, Hong LE. 2014. Neurodevelopmental and neurodegenerative models of schizophrenia: White matter at the centre stage. Schizophrenia Bulletin 40: 721-728.

Lambert T 2010 Targeting treatment refractory schizophrenia: A multidimensional outcome approach to the diagnosis and management of incomplete recovery. Australian Consensus Panel for Treatment-Refractory schizophrenia. www.trsconsensus.com.au

Large MM, Nielssen O. 2011 Violence in first episode psychosis: A systematic review and meta-analysis Schizophrenia Research125: 209-220.

Lopez LV and Kane JM. Plasma levels of second-generation antipsychotics and clinical response in acute psychosis: A review of the literature. Schizophrenia Research 2013. 147: 368-374

Marcelis M, Murray R et al. Urbanisation and psychosis: a study of 1942-1978 birth cohort in the Netherlands Psychol Med; 28: 871-879 1998.

McGorry, Yung et al. Randomised controlled trial of interventions designed to reduce the risk of progression to first episode psychosis in clinical sample with sub threshold symptoms. Arch Gen Psychiatry 2002; 59, 921-928.

Mendhkar ND. Hyperpigmentation with amisulpride ANZJP Volume 43, Number1, Jan 2009 page 88.

Mergui J, Jawarowski S et al. Shared OCD: Broadening the Concept of Shared Psychotic disorder ANZJP. Vol 44 No (9) 2010) 859-862.

Miles H, Miles N et al. Obstructive sleep apnoea and schizophrenia: a systematic review to inform clinical practice. Schizophrenia Res 2016; 170: 222-225.

Mortensen PB, Pederson CB, et al. Effects of family history and place and season of birth on the risk of schizophrenia. New Engl J Med 1999; 340: 603-608.

Mulder R, Rucklidge J, et al 2017. Why has increased provision of psychiatric treatment not reduced the prevalence of mental disorders? ANZJP 51:1173-1174

Nilsson E, Hultman CM, et al Schizophrenia and offspring's risk for adverse pregnancy outcomes and infant death. Br J Psychiatry 2008;193:311-315.

Pekala, E and Merinder, L.2002 Psycho-education for schizophrenia. Cochrane Data-base Systematic Review.

Ranning A, Laursen TM, et al. 2015 Serious mental illness and disrupted care giving for children. Journal of Clinical Psychiatry 76: e106-e1014.

Review of mental health services in Australia 2003-2008. Consumer and carer direct experiences of care. www.mhca.com.au/Consumer Care Survey 000.html).

Ross BM, Seguin J, et al.-3 fatty acid as treatment for mental illness: which disorder and which fatty acid? Lipid Health Dis. 2007; 6: 21.

Scott KM, de Jong P, et al. 2018 Discussion In: Mental Disorders Around the World: Facts and Figures from the WHO World Mental Health Survey. Cambridge: Cambridge University Press pp 324-336.

Scott J, Chant D et al. Association between trauma exposure and delusional experiences in large community-based sample. Br J Psychiatry 2007; 190: 339-343.

Slade M. Personal recovery and mental illness: a guide for mental health professionals. Cambridge University Press, 2009.

St Clair D, Xu M, et al. Rates of adult schizophrenia following prenatal exposure to the Chinese famine of 1959-1961 JAMA 2005; 294: 557-562.

Strawn JR, Kek PE, et al. Neuroleptic malignant syndrome Am J Psychiatry. 2007. 164: 870-876.

Susser ES Lin S. Schizophrenia after prenatal exposure to Dutch hunger winter 1944-1945. Arch Gen Psych 1992; 49: 983-988.

Tully J, Lally J, et al. 2016 Augmentation of clozapine with electroconvulsive therapy in treatment resistant schizophrenia: A systematic review and meta-analysis. Schizophrenia Research 171:215-224

Van Os J, Kenis G, et al. 2010 The environment and schizophrenia. Nature 468: 203-212.

Vita A, DePeri L, et al. 2015 The effect of antipsychotic treatment on cortical grey matter changes in schizophrenia: Does the class matter? A meta-analysis and meta-regression of longitudinal magnetic resonance imaging studies. Biological Psychiatry 78: 403-412.

Wan MW, Salmon MP, et al 2007 What predicts poor mother infant reaction in schizophrenia? Psychological Medicine 37:537-546.

Zhang TH, Xu LeeHua, et al. Real world effectiveness of antipsychotic treatment, in psychosis prevention in a 3 years cohort of 517 individuals, at clinical (ultra) high risk from the Shanghai. At Risk for Psychosis ANZJP May 2020.

MOODS DISORDER (AFFECTIVE DISORDER)

AFFECTIVE DISORDERS: ARE severe and recurring psychiatric conditions, with early onset and lifelong course, affecting 1-3% of global population and sixth leading cause of disability among all diseases (Whiteford et al. 2010). These are a group of illnesses with the two principal diagnostic categories being bipolar disorder and major depressive disorder. Major depressive episodes are central feature of both.

"It has profound impact on social and economic mobility in addition to, untold personal suffering. I am now the most miserable man living. If what I feel were equally distributed to the whole human family, there will not be one cheerful face on this earth. Whether I shall ever be better, I cannot tell; I awfully forbade I should not. To remain as I am is impossible; I must die or be better."

Abraham Lincoln, personal correspondence to family lawyer 1842.

Depression

Depression is common mental disorder, with an estimated 350 million people, of all ages affected worldwide. With lifetime prevalence of 16%, major depressive disorders have been identified as, the leading cause of disability and global burden around the world, after ischemic heart disease, according to, WHO survey. Taken together with anxiety, it is the largest single cause of disability among both men and women in Australia and responsible for nearly 20% of lived with disability years.

On average, those who were able to remain in workforce as the result of prevention of depression would earn between $28,000 and $48,000 more per year, and net government revenues would increase by around $ 5 million (Veerman2005).

It has comorbid relationship with heart disease, cancer, stroke, obesity, diabetes and arthritis to name a few.

Case Study

I first met him when he was 14 years olds. He was the only son of two professional teachers and, a brother of 3 sisters. He was a compliant, intelligent and good-natured boy, in a close-knit family. His school grades were high, though he was gradually losing interest in his peer group, and isolating himself for the past several months. He was quieter at home and seemed unhappy for no obvious reason. His appetite was diminished with no change in his body weight. Apart from the schoolwork, he preferred to sleep. Although he felt worthless, there was no suicidal thought. He was seen by the school counselor, and than by a local psychologist. Due to his young age his general practitioner was reluctant to prescribe any medication. So the challenge was in my hands. I started with anti-depressant medication and talk therapy. He was a likeable boy with glimpse of vision beyond his depression. So we worked well together, though not without the peaks and troughs, and we both determined to see, as what lies beyond his depression. I saw his parents with and without him. There were periods when he remained well, and did not see me for months. After finishing his HSC he went to Ireland to visit his extended family, which I reassured him was a positive step, towards his recovery. I was unfortunately wrong. He was hospitalized in UK following a massive overdose, and his father rushed to bring him home. I kept him in the hospital, where I was a VMO, for another fortnight. He made good progress enrolled himself at the university in an arts degree and met his first girlfriend. Despite his long periods of remissions, the trauma of his lost years of life, never allowed him to fully recover. Towards the end of his graduation, he decided, to take yet another challenge, to prove himself. I was excited for him when he shared with me the plan to do medicine. It set a new agenda for us to work together. He started preparing for Graduate Medical School Admissions Test (GMSAT). As the time for his examination was approaching, his depression started to get worse, resisting most of the interventions and requiring hospitalization. He had responded to electroconvulsive therapy in the past, though I was reluctant to consider it, due to its effect on the cognitive functions even in short term. After consulting my colleagues, I finally decided to try it as the last resort. More than anyone, I was keen for him to attempt the examination, though he was in the hospital. His parents accepted his inability to proceed, if he could not attempt the examination, but agreed to drive him to Sydney University on the day. I gave him longer interval between his 6th and 7th treatment and he gathered hope and drive, for yet another challenge.

It was a long admission for him, though all his losses seemed to recover when he got the news of his success. He casually worked through his graduation to financially support himself, and we met frequently to review his medication, which was all he required. He steadily climbed the ladder moving to work in various hospitals of NSW and then went to Melbourne. Our last contact was when he informed me that he changed his mind, from doing psychiatry as his post graduation, to anesthesiology. I warmed up to our joint accomplished mission.

It has not been only a lesson but reinforced my belief, that there is more to human health, and recovery from illness, beyond the prescriptions. Human mind is the strongest determinant of success. He had a goal, a dream, and light at the end of the tunnel: he could see with hope, energizing him, and motivating him to continue driving.

Until the outset of 20th century, psychiatry was primarily based on extreme forms of mental illnesses, which resulted in social and oppressive measures to control it. This may have been the reason for the paucity of literature on depression, also known as neurasthenia or melancholy. A Treatise of Melancholy by Timothy Bright in 1586, and Anatomy of Melancholia published in 1620 were, some of the earliest books on the subject. The milestone was erected in 1899 with the publication of scientific treatise, "Depression: What It Is and How to Cure It" by AE Bridger, making the transition to new outlook, from the antiquity of impaired body fluids, like black bile.

Depression, the most frequently diagnosed mental disorder of 21st century, also a common word, to describe any upset: is undermining its seriousness as an illness. As a clinical diagnosis, it is nearly incomprehensible for anyone who has not experienced it in its extreme mode.

After nearly 200 years of history, depression has yet to find its discerning identity not to be confused with normal emotion of depression. Its journey from neurasthenia and melancholia, through depression, major depressive disorder, mood disorder, affective disorder and now bipolar disorder have been destabilizing. If that was not enough Akiskal in 1999 described 9 subtypes of bipolar disorders ranging from half (schizobipolar) to bipolar IV (depression with hyper-thymic temperament, or trait hypomania) (Akiscal HS, etal.1999).

'I got so low that I asked to be hospitalised and for deep narcosis (sleep). I cannot stand being awake. The pain is too much— something has happened to me, this vital spark has stopped burning-I go to dinner table now and I don't say a word, just sit there like a Dodo. Normally I am the center of attention, keep the conversation going-so that is distressing me'

"Anonymous"

Diagnostic criteria for depressive disorder

Depressive disorder has the usual feature of anhedonia (loss of pleasure), accompanied by psychomotor disturbances like changes in weight, fatigue, sleep disturbance, cognitive symptoms, hopelessness, guilt, suicidal thoughts and helplessness etc.

Major depressive disorder has subcategories like Persistent; depression disorder.

Disruptive mood, dysregulation disorder for children with frequent outbursts of anger and persistent irritability.

Premenstrual: dysphoric, disorder.

Substance /medication induced depressive disorder. Depressive disorder, due to another, medical condition.

Most of the medical conditions are likely to cause reactive, if not endogenous/biological depression. It is the most common psychiatric disorder in epilepsy, both with controlled and uncontrolled seizures. There are psycho-social as well as biological factors like hypo-metabolism in extra-temporal regions. The interictal, and dysphoric disorders may include, more atypical symptoms like anxiety, bipolar, somatoform, anergia, pain, fear etc of possible longer duration.

Seemingly irreversible mental disorders, and dementia might in fact be masked depression, which the psychiatrist should be mindful of.

BIPOLAR DISORDER

OUR TRAINING INCLUDED manic–depressive psychosis, which was renamed bipolar disorder in 1980 in DSM-3.

It constitutes a severe mental disorder generally manifesting, during late adolescence or early adulthood. It has progressive course characterised by, inter-episodic periods of euthymia, without full functional or cognitive recovery. Poor sustained attention, deficits in executive functions, learning and memory can get it confused, with ADHD in early stages. Cognitive functioning may worsen with multiple episodes.

Early recognition and early treatment are vitally important, as executive functions mediated by the frontal lobes, continue to develop from childhood in to late adolescents and early adulthood (Samame C, et al. 2014).

Identification of risk factors (bipolar prodrome) may help to minimise the illness or its serious negative consequences. Personality, temperament and character traits, sleep and circadian rhythm may be modifiable risk factors. The time of puberty and adolescence is generally marked by significant emotional and social developmental changes, which makes it difficult to differentiate between healthy and pathological features. It is important to watch for the duration, intensity and its impact on the subject. Childhood anxiety, impaired emotional regulation, hypersensitivity, somatic complaints, excessive guilt, inability to find pleasure, long periods of depressed or elated mood and diurnal variations need to be followed up. In addition to this, poor sleep quality in a young person also carries a risk (Pfennig A, et al. 2017).

So, the staging, which sets the trajectory; begins with family history of genetic endowment, early non specific risk syndrome, via childhood risk syndromes regarding anxiety and sleep, to the onset of minor and later major depressive disorder, before the appearance of diagnosable bipolar disorder. It is equally important to identify the potential resilience factors to remain healthy. Life style behaviour, physical activity, quality of social and interpersonal interactions, and ability of coping with stress, are likely to counteract some of the risk factors.

Diagnostic Criteria

The turbulence commenced, with the introduction of bipolar 2 disorders in DSM-4, which identified it, as of lesser severity, and arbitrary boundaries, open to misuse and misdiagnosis. I have met many self-diagnosed young people convinced of their bipolar diagnosis to justify their antisocial or unacceptable behaviour. The close boundary of bipolar-2 with normal mood is, likely to cause missed or over-diagnosis. Both bipolar 1 and bipolar 2 share the same treatment, which, can also be questionable in the expansion of bipolar spectrum disorders. Although it remains debatable both are included in DSM V and ICD.

If these 2 confounding subcategories were not enough, the bipolar-3 was introduced, though not included in DSM-5, which is treatment emergent affective switch. It is thought to represent the unmasking of underlying bipolar diathesis or spontaneous mania. This occurs against the background of recurring episodes of depression in context of antidepressant treatment and the periods of hypomania are brief.

At least one manic episode is followed or preceded, by a, depressive episode.

Diagnosis is made difficult due to confounding factors.

Bipolar illness is a recurring illness, with a lifelong course: between threshold and sub-threshold symptoms. Despite modern guidelines, concordant and evidence based pharmacotherapy and psychotherapy, only about 30% patients achieve sustained wellness (Perlis RH, et al.2006).

Bipolar disorder generally begins with depressive episodes, before developing mania (hypo). Lifetime prevalence of unipolar depression is 10 – 15 times higher than bipolar disorder (STEP-BD 2006).

Cognitive impairment in mood disorders has been recognized for many years, specially, in elderly, where it has been described as, pseudo-dementia. It is therefore essential to consider organic differential diagnoses. Unfortunately some cognitive impairment remains even during the part remission periods.

Based on pathophysiology, there has been continuous search to identify biomarkers to refine the diagnosis of bipolar disorders. Immune dysfunction, alterations in oxidative stress parameters, neuroplasticity, peripheral changes in cytokines, the content of lipid peroxidation, oxidative damage to proteins and neuro-trophic factors have been consistently associated with mood disorders (Pfaffenseller B, et al. 2013). A recent study showed that severity of depression, number of episodes and suicidal attempts are associated with activated immune and oxidative pathways, which can be a promising diagnostic tool, to potentially aid the clinical assessment of mood disorders and current suicidal ideation. (Sowa-Kucma M, et al. 2018).

Mixed Mood-States: Psychomotor agitation and fatigue or loss of energy can be useful in differentiating whether the predominant mood state and context of the mixed symptoms are that of mania or depression, respectively. Mixed mood states can be separated clinically into Mixed Mania and Mixed Depression on the basis of psychomotor activity and energy (Malhi 2015).

Melancholia: is defined as non reactive and anhedonic depressed mood, lack of energy, foggy concentration and diurnal mood variation, as well as psychomotor disturbances which are also shared with other depressive disorders. Melancholia's descriptions include, set of distinctive clinical features, genetic, rather than psychosocial determinants, biological underpinning, a minimal response to placebo and a preferential response to medication and ECT than to psychotherapy (Parker G 2017).

The term pseudo-melancholia was, coined by Prof G. Parker of University of NSW, to highlight the possibility of misdiagnosis and delayed treatment. Many neurological and neurodegenerative disorders can mimic the presentation of melancholia; at least in the initial stages. Most of the dementing illnesses as well as multiple sclerosis and brain injuries like haematoma can induce depressed mood and psychomotor disturbances eclipsing the diagnosis of underlying organic disease (Parker, G. 2020).

Case Study

A 42 years old divorced man with 3 children, who worked as a builder. He was transferred under my care from his retiring psychiatrist. He had earlier episodes of severe depression dating back to age 30 years. He required multiple hospital admissions the previous year, in quick succession, with suicidal thoughts and grievous body injuries. There was significant marital disharmony and financial difficulties prevailing at the time, beyond his capacity to resolve. He lost insight, became noncompliant, and severely distressed, as the marriage continued to deteriorate. Feeling helpless and despondent: he shot himself with a gun, inflicting serious abdominal injuries, requiring life support, laparotomy, recto-sigmoid resection, bladder repair and colostomy in 2003.

He was resistant to most available treatments including ECT.

He was older of 2 boys. His father operated a small though successful business. The family lived on their farm in semi rural setting. His mother was diagnosed with schizophrenia. He remembered many occasions, much to his distress, when she needed involuntary hospitalisations, being taken by police and ambulance from their home. The family environment was impacted by his father's business commitments, and mother's illness. During his adolescent years, he suffered from bouts of self-resolving depressive episodes. He did not require treatment till his first admission at the age of 30 years. His brother left home, venturing out in the world of illicit drugs, for which he was, disowned by the family.

When he came under my care he was pursuing with a business course at the local technical college. He separated from his wife and lost custody of his 3 children. He was still grieving for the loss. He was living on the farm, with his animals. His father was placed in a nursing home following his wife's death in 2005 as he was suffering from worsening dementia.

He had a fluctuating course of depression, though with periods of remission, when he functioned well. He started a new relationship, which was supportive, and he started to build his hopes for a family life. They had a child, giving him new life, as he did not see his older children, since the family break-up. Unfortunately it had the same fate as before, losing even the visiting access to his son. He felt increasingly despondent and was often not able to go to work.

After an hour-long session with me one evening in 2011, he suddenly left without conclusion of our session. For the next hour he did not respond to my repeated phone calls. I then informed the local police with my grave fear. The land and air search began after announcing on the local radio, which alerted him. He hid under his bed before jumping into the river, which flows through his property: remaining under water. After over an hour he was spotted by a helicopter and taken to hospital.

I referred him in 2015 to a senior colleague for second opinion, for the possibility of treating him with a psycho-stimulant in long term, having started it earlier. In agreement, with and approval of the consultant, he continued on dexamphetamine with authority prescriptions. We discussed at length the possibility of dependence and other relevant adverse effects of long-term use of dexamphetamine. He finally responded to the medication though not exceeding 15 mg a day. He subsequently went to Vietnam for a holiday with a friend who introduced him to his future wife. He stayed in the country for 3 months and revisited a few times before marrying. The couple had 3 daughters. The stable family life gave him the missing link though he continued to take dexamphetamine, resistant to the idea of withdrawal.

He worked on the farm, made an impressive model aircraft and worked as bricklayer, for 6 years after starting the dexamphetamine, and 7 years since his last admission.

There were subclinical symptoms of brief elated mood at the verge of grandiosity, overvalued ideas, immature fantasies, sense of persecution and outlandish imagery, which pointed towards weak genetic endowment possibly inherited from his mother. Nevertheless the symptoms remained sub-threshold and he was able to function at a reasonable level with minimal reservation.

This case emphasizes that the basic knowledge in psychiatry needs to be shaped uniquely around each patient, not to our expectations but to patient's maximum potential and functional reality.

Aetiology

The evolution of neurotransmitter hypothesis, underlying mood disorder was exciting, and led to the discovery of first and second generation of antidepressants. It remains the most validated base of aetiology and pathophysiology.

Research evidence is now exploring the relationship, between depression and inflammation, which may not be a new idea. Brain inflammation was believed as the root of insanity. The use of humoral therapies for maladies, were common practice worldwide in the 17th and 18th centuries.

The current hypothesis is that, depression is associated with, low-grade inflammation indicated by, higher concentration of C-reactive protein, interleukin-6 and tumour necrosis factor, well above their healthy counterparts (Haapacoski, et al.2015). Inflammation has particular relevance, as it can influence many physiological disturbances, implicated in depression, such as neurotransmitter activities, HPA axis activity, oxidative and nitrosative stress, mitochondrial activity and neuro-progression (Moylan et al 2013).

The causes of subclinical inflammation are considered multifactorial, comprising biological psychological, social and lifestyle factors.

Current and past stress and trauma can influence, the immune response. History of childhood abuse and trauma is a risk factor, for higher inflammation. Acute and chronic stressors also influence the inflammatory response. Stress and its resulting high cortisol level, can impair CNS and peripheral nervous system feedback, leading to glucocorticoid resistance and impairment of mitochondrial function (Rodriguez et al 2016). This impacts on gut microbiome and ultimately compromising the immune response.

Eating unhealthy diet, poor sleep and reduced physical activity are associated with increased inflammation.

The physical conditions like obesity, diabetes, cardiovascular and digestive disorders and autoimmune diseases are also associated with increased inflammation (Riparelia et al 2015).

There is increasing evidence of the role of pro-inflammatory cytokines,-a family of protein, that mediate immune responses to injury, infections and other organismal stresses, as well as synaptic transmission, neuroplasticity and neuroendocrine regulation. These are raised in both serum and CSF of the patients with depressive disorders (Young et al 2014). This has led to the importance of inflammation in many psychiatric disorders like schizophrenia, mood disorders, PTSD, autism and anxiety disorders.

There has been reported effectiveness of anti-inflammatory and immune modulatory drugs, such as aspirin and celecoxib, used as adjunctive treatment, in psychiatric disorders including schizophrenia and depression (Muller N.2019). Therefore there is need for objective and accurate measure of the inflammation, which can be achieved by neutrophil-lymphocyte ratio (NLR), calculated by dividing neutrophil count by lymphocyte count. Neutrophil forms an important part of innate immune system, plays a prominent role in bacterial infections and often the first responders to tissue inflammation. Lymphocytes include natural killer cells, T cells and B cells, typically elevated with viral infections, and form core of the adaptive immune system (Zlatan Zulfic. 2020).

NLR is dynamic and is influenced by inflammatory cytokines and endocrine effects of the hypothalamic pituitary adrenal axis. Generally both acute and chronic inflammations cause elevated NLR through a relative neutrophilia and lymphopenia. NLR correlates with C-reactive protein levels in patients with psychosis, which can be used with much less cost and more convenience. NLR could predict treatment response and outcome in psychiatry. Elevated NLR has been found in many psychiatric conditions. However its projected role in, psychiatry, remains limited pending more research in the area.

More recently gut microbial composition has been associated with number of illnesses, including psychiatric disorders (Moya, et al 2016), which is a promising theory. Gut microbe is a dynamic entity, influenced by several factors like genetics, diet, metabolism, age, antibiotic treatment and stress.

Major Depressive disorder has been associated with, reduction in microbial richness and diversity, as well as changes in relative abundance of specific microbial taxa (Winter G, et al 2018). Activation of immune system by the gut microbes was proposed as the key pathway in the gut brain axis, impacting on behavioural changes. Abnormal immune activation as a pivotal pathophysiological mechanism, in bipolar disorder has been reported in several studies (Passos IC, et al 2015).

Immune activation is likely to become potential therapeutic target, as well as marker of treatment response in bipolar disorders.

Due to differences in the individual microbial and the antimicrobial effect of antidepressants, there may be interpersonal variability in treatment efficacy. This may also develop into routine assessment for, drug efficacy in the future (McGovern A, et al. 2019).

There is mounting evidence of limbic system: the neural counterpart, being responsible for the emotional processing. BPAD has strong neurobiological basis that involves dysfunction of anterior limbic brain network.

Among structural brain changes are; reduced hippocampal volume and grey matter alterations in prefrontal region, specially anterior cingulate cortex and medial frontal regions (Bora E, et al 2012) Smaller hippocampal volume is possibly associated with chronic depression, longer course of illness, number of recurrent episodes and early onset of depression (McMaster FP, et al 2004).

The role of amygdala is important; as its hyperactivity is related to negative emotions and reduced volume, to genetic risk factor. There are some studies suggestive of brain changes before the onset of depression: a predisposition and trait factor for the disorder.

The volume of stress sensitive structures such as hippocampus is reported to be highly genetically determined with heritability rate as high as 80% (Glahen DC, et al. 2012).

Environmental risk factors specially, childhood maltreatment, also appear to alter limbic and prefrontal brain structures in healthy subjects similar to findings in MDD patients (Opel N, et al. 2014).

Neurotoxicity hypothesis states, that acute depression initiates neurobiological changes that in turn lead to extended activation of hypothalamic pituitary adrenal (HPA) axis, resulting in prolonged and repeated cortisol release, consequently hyper-cortisolism leads to decreased neurogenesis. Hippocampal atrophy is associated with time spent in untreated depressive state and such morphometric marker resolves with antidepressant medication or ECT, both of which cause hippocampal neurogenesis, with associated larger hippocampal volume. (Dukart J, et al. 2014). Remission stops the increased cortisol levels, which in turn prevents continued damage to brain structures. In contrast, non-remitted patients experience, further toxic cortisol release with, reduction in stress sensitive hippocampal volume and more brain atrophy.

The gradual brain atrophy is now a well-known feature of ageing. Therefore depression after the age of 65 years, may share brain pathology of ageing brain.

Bipolar disorders more than unipolar are viewed as one of the most heritable disorders, estimated at nearly 10 times that of general population. The advancement in genetics has been exploring role of genes in mood disorders. The current hypothesis is that the mood disorders occur in a genetically predisposed individual and are triggered by exposure to deleterious environmental factors, which can change the activity of biochemical pathway through the modulation of epigenetic mechanism (Craddock N 2006).

Neuropsychological symptoms including depression often result from neurological, psychological or just part of ageing like apathy of cognitive impairment causing diagnostic dilemma. There can be co-morbid neurological, neurodegenerative or psychiatric disorders impacting on diagnosis, treatment or progression of the disease.

There has been progress in objective criteria to diagnose psychiatric illnesses, which hopefully will improve the diagnosis, eliminating the confounding factors.

Organic Mania (Psychosis)

Colloid cyst of third ventricle may present with variety of psychiatric symptoms, including chronic mania, with persistence of manic symptoms without remission over a long period of time (Uvais NA et al. 2020) The cases reported in the literature resolved completely after surgical intervention (Javed Q, 2014)

Although uncommon, it can result from focal brain lesions and other neurological conditions, as well as cerebrovascular diseases. Symptoms of organic mania can be overwhelming, over and above the organic illness, which can be easily missed. Therefore one needs to be, aware of its atypical presentation of late onset, no family or previous history of affective symptoms, and some indication of physical, specially, neurological and cerebrovascular symptoms. Mania may overshadow, other aspects of clinical presentation, which can easily be overlooked.

Corticosteroid induced mania has been known since its discovery in 1949. Manic or hypomanic symptoms can appear, within hours of starting the drug. Additionally there is increased risk of depression and higher risk of delirium, after its discontinuation. DSM 5 has described it as medication induced bipolar disorder. Co-administration of drugs, which are P450 CYP 3A4 inhibitor that inhibits, the breakdown of prednisone and its active metabolites, have been shown to predispose to mania. Elderly patients are more prone to corticosteroid complications such as depression, delirium, mania, confusion and disorientation.

Autoimmune-Encephalitis: Associated with antibodies against NMDA receptors, can present with neuropsychiatric symptoms after 2 weeks of nonspecific prodromal symptoms. Catatonia, with intermittent agitation and excitation, mutism, and global cognitive impairment, may direct the patient to a psychiatrist. However rapid onset of first episode of psychiatric symptoms followed by seizures, abnormal involuntary movements and extrapyramidal symptoms must alert the examiner for the possibility of organic aetiology. In older patients it has been reported to resemble diffuse neurodegenerative disease. Diagnosis is made by, testing of NMDAR antibodies in plasma, and CSF. Early diagnosis and treatment, with immunotherapy or surgery, if required, caries favourable prognosis (Pruss H et al 2017).

Pregnancy and bipolar disorder

Reproductive cycle events like menstrual-cycle, pregnancy, postnatal period and menopause may impact on the course of illness for women with bipolar disorder. Some women have greater propensity of mood worsening of mood symptoms at each of these reproductive cycle events. The risk factors for it are likely to be earlier age of onset of mood symptoms and comorbid anxiety, rapid cycling, history of self-harm and mixed mood presentation.

Interaction between oestrogen, progesterone, brain derived neuro-trophic factor, oxidative stress and inflammation pathways may be particularly relevant for women with bipolar disorder, which is the potential mechanism for increased risk of relapse (Frey 2014). Pre and postnatal period as well as pregnancy, are well documented times for recurrence of symptoms specially, with relapse risk for those, who cease medication during pregnancy. The symptom emergence is rapid in the final week of pregnancy, and early in post partum. There are risks involved both short and long term for the foetus and the baby. Prophylactic lithium has been effective. However judicious use of medication is recommended, as there may be potential risk to the foetus and the infant. Psychological treatment, remain first line of intervention.

Maternal anxiety, stress and depression have significant impact on the outcome both for the mother and the child. Untreated ante and postnatal depression have been associated with poor language development, lower IQ in adolescence and developmental delay (Deave T, et al. 2008).

Treatment

It was not till late 1950s when the serious research on the neurobiology, began highlighting the dysfunction of CNS, subserved by monoamine transmitters. Subsequently MAOI and tricyclics were introduced into psychiatry in 1957, transforming the entire domain of mental illnesses forever.

Failure to respond for a depressed patient is more common, than responding, which can be blamed on the complexity of its diagnosis, as depression is the reaction to any unwanted unpleasantness, or psychosocial stressor, apart from being of endogenous origin, with no perceptible or obvious reason. At least 10% of patients initially diagnosed with unipolar depression, will subsequently experience mania/hypomania in the course of their illness, resulting in revision of their diagnosis to bipolar disorder, and the modification of therapy usually involving the addition of a mood stabilizer (Fiedorowicz JG, et al.2011).

Desired response of only one third of patients, with initial antidepressant treatment; is a significant issue in managing depression.

Treatment of bipolar affective disorder was much simpler when I started my training. Manic depression was treated with tricyclic antidepressants or lithium. Over the past 2 decades it seems to have become more complex and controversial with no indisputable, consistent guidelines till the publication of Clinical Practice Guidelines of RANZCP. I was most impressed with the 128 pages of the guidelines for mood disorders published by RANZCP after exhaustive and comprehensive review of world literature on affective disorders under the leadership of Prof Gin Malhi. The document, spanning for nearly 3 years of preparation, includes expert reviews as well as public consultations, is almost like a textbook. It addresses broad based conceptual issues, as well as everyday practical concerns. The combination of both evidence based and consensus-based viewpoints have heightened its clinical and educational utility. It has been widely applauded to the extent of describing it as an easy step-by-step tool-box for daily practice (Geoffray PA2016). The only criticism seems to be the consideration of cost in the choice of treatment like TMS or psychotherapy.

I specially liked the introductory paragraph that 'effective clinical care involves the art of applying clinical knowledge and skills; to the individual needs of those presenting for care'.

Australia ranked as second largest consumer of antidepressants, among 23 countries reported, and yet its use in bipolar depression is fiercely debated.

Prescribing off label antidepressants is widely practiced which may add to the high number of prescriptions. SSRIs are largely used for mental illnesses, and tricyclic for physical conditions like pain, migraine and urinary incontinence. In 2011, 89 defined daily dosages of antidepressants were dispensed per 1000 people (WHO, 2012).

Being a female, and lower level of education, income and health, were associated with higher use of antidepressants: was the conclusion of a large population based cohort study from NSW Australia (Paige E, et al. 2015). Low cost access to subsidised medication was given one of the reasons for its excessive use.

Some studies have claimed that conventional antidepressants may worsen the course of bipolar disorders exacerbating mood instability though it has been refuted (Sidor MM, et al.2011)

The expectation of the treatment is to reduce the symptoms, by 50% during the acute phase. It should continue to improve till the remission stage, which takes about 6 weeks leading to residual symptoms and signs. This is followed by recovery to premorbid stage, and thereafter maintenance to prevent recurrence, and enhance resilience. Ideally the goal of the success should involve, the collaborative plan of, the expertise of the clinician, and the other health care professionals involved, as well as lived experience of the patient, family, carer and the support group.

Despite the controversies and no reliable predictor of response to medication or choice of it, antidepressants are still recommended as first line treatment for adults with moderate to severe depression. It comes as no surprise, that at least half of the people diagnosed with moderate degree of depression, and are likely to benefit from its use, and yet do not use antidepressants (Harris MG, et al. 2015).

The prescribing should be based on side effect profile, tolerability, cost, suicide risk, clinician's experience and the intensity of depression. There is mounting evidence suggesting potential link between antidepressant use and range of adverse events like mortality, fractures, cardiovascular events and gastrointestinal and intracranial bleeding (Coupland C, et al 2018).

It is estimated that approximately, 6% of men and 17% of women suffer from osteoporosis in Australia leading to increased incidence of fractures. An often overlooked, contributory factor to bone fragility is depression itself. A growing body of evidence suggests that depression and schizophrenia are associated with low bone mineral density or increased bone loss over time (Moura C. 2014). Well-known risk factors shared by, psychiatric disorders and osteoporosis, include alcohol and substance abuse, smoking, inactivity, stress, sleep deprivation, poor eating habits, vitamin D deficiency, genetic factors and medications like glucocorticoids. The psychotropic medications with deleterious effect on bone include valproate, carbamazepine, sertraline and fluoxetine, along with, many antipsychotic drugs (Williams LJ 201`6).

The risk of osteoporosis should be taken into account when prescribing antidepressants.

Therefore antidepressants should not be routinely used to treat sub-threshold or mild depression, as the benefit may not outweigh the potential risk.

An adequate trial at recommended therapeutic dose of antidepressant should be minimum of 3 weeks.

In Australia GPs prescribe 70% of antidepressants for depression, 16% for other psychological problems and 10% for musculoskeletal, neurological and menstrual problems. Some may also continue to prescribe at the request of patients who only benefit from its placebo effect. There should be a review at the time of renewing the prescription for the necessity of its continuation.

There is no significant difference in the efficacy between tricyclic and newer generation of antidepressants, apart from the safety profile in favour of the new generation antidepressants, which also have safety issues. There has been adverse publicity of emergence or worsening suicidal thoughts, with SSRI in the first few weeks. So it is important to monitor all patients during the first month.

The introduction of traditional anti-convalescents and atypical neuroleptics in line with lithium are, increasingly recognized mood stabilizers, replacing conventional antidepressants. For most patients with depression, a combination treatment approach is more effective than either psychological or antidepressant treatment alone. For this reason, co-prescription of medications, from different classes, is common. Most commonly prescribed antidepressants inhibit hepatic cytochrome P450 enzymes that metabolises most of the psychotropic drugs, creating the potential for pharmacokinetic drug interactions leading to increased plasma concentration and possible toxicity.

If the psychodynamic formulation of mood disorder was enchanting for me, the neurobiological revelations are almost spellbound. The oldest and humble mood-stabilizer lithium has never ceased to amaze the scientists. Psychiatry started to change in 1949 after the introduction of lithium, and was followed by discoveries of neuroleptics and antidepressants. Although John Cade, an Australian psychiatrist, is widely associated with Lithium: it was used in ancient Greece for mental disorders, and in late 19th century, by others, for mental disorders as well as nature's antidote, for liquor and opium habit. Lithium is the lightest and oldest metal. Trace amounts are found in human body. It may be involved in a variety of physiological processes.

There is evidence that bipolar disorders are associated with brain ageing, disproportionately to chronological ageing, as well as with increased risk of dementia. There is also sufficient evidence to support the neuro-protective role of lithium, in the mechanism involved in accelerated ageing, and neuro-progression (Hajek T, et al 2016). It is protective against white and grey matter loss and promotes neuronal regeneration.

It improves, cognition, mood and brain structures, reduces oxidative stress and has anti-suicidal effect, beyond mood stabilisation (Malhi GS, et al. 2013).

Lithium is the only psychotropic drug, which, enhances bone integrity and reduces fractures (Liu B, et al 2019).

Its effectiveness as an augmenting agent, by exerting synergistic antidepressant effect, has been strongly supported by randomized controlled trials. Lithium remains the gold standard; although it has been through phases, when it was overtaken by newer drugs, albeit temporarily. Nevertheless with available choice of multiple mood stabilisers, lithium may not be the first line of treatment, due to its slow onset of action in acute mania and less effective in acute bipolar depression. Although lithium appears to meet the definition of true mood stabiliser, its chronic therapeutic administration, needs careful monitoring of thyroid and parathyroid glands, as well as of renal functions for possible end stage renal diseases. Cardiovascular complications of lithium can occur, independent of the therapeutic level, and the duration of treatment. However its effect on heart is reversible once it is withdrawn. Therefore ECG monitoring is recommended (Yu et al. 2015).

According to Ethno-Psychopharmacology: an evolving branch, there are ethnic variations and familial patterns influencing the effectiveness of psychotropic medications. Some ethnic groups have higher rates of rapid metaboliser status, at the hepatic cytochrome P450 enzyme system, requiring higher doses of medication.

Noncompliance of prescribed treatment may not be deliberate but it causes disturbance in the continuity of progress. World Health organization has reported that 50% of patients from developed countries with chronic disease do not use their medications as recommended. Low adherence with any prescribed treatment is very common (Horn R. et al. 2006).

Bipolar Affective Disorder (BAD) like any other chronic illness requires long-term prophylaxis to prevent recurrences. The reasons for noncompliance may be varied apart from tolerability, undesirable side effects and unconvincing role of medication. Rate of relapse in BAD is as high as 40% irrespective of the compliance in the first year, 60% in the second year, and 73% over five years or more. (Gitlin M, et-al. 1995).

Psychosocial contributors and interventions to noncompliance must be considered, to address the issues. Self-monitoring and family involvement in decision making are useful strategies in enforcing compliance.

Managing manic symptoms can be more challenging, as it can be complicated by factors, like depression, anxiety or substance abuse. It is also associated with marked behavioural and cognitive disturbance with psychosis, occurring in 60% cases during acute episodes (Malhi et al 2009). Manic symptoms can occur within depression, as mixed features, with increasing severity from hypomania and mania, and through to mania with psychosis.

Pharmacological anti-manic agents have a relatively modest response rates, in the short duration of standard trials. For quick symptomatic control of behaviour, benzodiazepines are used for short period, followed by anti manic, anti-convalescent, and antipsychotic drugs as indicated. Combined mood stabilizer and antipsychotic treatment is more effective, as first line of treatment than mono-therapy with either. For severe or high risk patients, ECT may be required.

The management of mood disorder is an individual (personalized) endeavour. It is important to understand the person, in the context of their unique circumstances. This is the cornerstone of successful therapeutic relationship.

There is mounting evidence of social and psychological therapies, to empower the individual, with coping and healing strategies. Resilience, social support and lifestyle changes are some, which can be delivered via cognitive reappraisal therapy.

Psychological Therapies

Adjunctive psychotherapy can be very beneficial as it targets the areas which medications do not address, such as teaching the individual about the illness, providing skills to control their mood fluctuations, coping with stressful life events, improving social rhythm, sleep patterns and interpersonal relationships.

Improved subjective quality of life, personal recovery, self-confidence and good therapeutic relationship, based on respect, support, empathy and warmth are all critical to optimal outcome. There is strong evidence of the role of psycho-education and psychotherapy in carer burnout. There is ever growing evidence base for psychodynamic psychotherapy, and a sustained and flourishing interest, in the application of psychodynamic theories, and practice alongside other treatments, to the care of wide variety of patients (Gilligan 2015).

Early findings from imaging studies have shown that some forms of psychotherapy and mindfulness result in significant changes in white matter and functional network efficiency of brain (Wang T 2013).

Therefore government has progressively invested large funds since 2006 in psychological treatment running at over AUD $28m per week for improving the quality of care (Sebastian R, et al.2019).

Research has now established that cognitive impairment; is a core feature of major depressive disorder, and that impairment persists even after clinical recovery. Its impact on day-to-day functioning in occupational and social situations is significant, which hinders full recovery. Therefore drug treatment should be complemented by cognitive enhancement/remediation therapy, which includes psycho-education, cognitive practice and its application in daily life to improve executive functions like working memory. Cognitive remediation may counteract maladaptive brain plasticity specially, in the early stages of depression when functional impairment may outweigh structural changes. The resulting neuro-plastic changes, increase brain activity in prefrontal cortex: known to be hypoactive in depression, improving cognitive deficit and depression (Snyder HR 2013).

Effective clinical communication is the key to any treatment. It leads to better health outcome, including higher satisfaction, improved illness understanding and adherence to treatment. Doctors have been often criticised for their poor communication skills. It was identified by RANZCP as core curriculum, Entrust-able Professional Activity: required for progression, through training.

In mild and moderate episodes of depression psychological management alone can be adequate. The real effect of psychotherapy specially, cognitive behavioural and interpersonal therapies is likely to be modest but not without value. With well-trained and experienced therapist the outcome of mild to moderate depression could be at the level of pharmacotherapy.

Cognitive Behavioural Therapy

It is possible that CBT instigates, positive lifestyle changes like improved sleep and diet etc, which impacts on the proposed theory of inflammation. CBT encourages formal relaxation techniques and pleasurable activities, which are protective against inflammation. Long-term CBT interventions may be associated with reduced body weight and increased glycaemic control specially, in patients, with obesity and diabetes. Such changes are associated with inflammation reduction over time (Lopresti 2013).

Antidepressant medication has been demonstrated to have anti-inflammatory effect postulating that reduced inflammation may be the potential mechanism behind their antidepressant effect (Hannestad. 2011).

Despite extensive evidence of effectiveness, cognitive behavioural therapy is difficult to access due to its cost and paucity of trained therapists. Therefore, computerised CBT has been an instant boon, embraced around the world enthusiastically: **Mood-GYM** developed by Australian National University is freely available internet-based programme for depression, which can be provided with or without clinician guidance (Twomey C, et al 2014). There is qualified support for the effectiveness of Mood-GYM from several randomised clinical trials: more for depression and to lesser extent for anxiety.

By combining the potentially stress reducing skills covered in CBT, the neurotransmitter effects of antidepressants and the anti-inflammatory influences of both treatments, a greater treatment response may be realised. Other options to consider include life style changes, targeting sleep, diet, yoga, meditation, mindfulness and exercise which all have potential anti-inflammatory influence.

There is robust evidence based support for, the inter-relationship between CBT and other psychological therapies, on the physiological processes implicated in depression. Mindfulness based cognitive therapy is a group based program that as an intervention, indicated for people with 3 or more previous major depressive episodes, has demonstrated efficacy in reducing relapse and recurrence (Segal et al 2002).

Brain Stimulation Therapy

Electro convulsive therapy (ECT) despite its chequered trajectory has maintained its place at least as the 2nd line of treatment specially, in treatment of resistant patients. Most recent theories of its mechanism of action relate to neurogenesis in the hippocampus.

It was developed, as the perceived theory of, biological antagonism between schizophrenia and epilepsy, by Cerletti & Bini in 1938. Hugh Birch built the first ECT machine in Adelaide Australia in 1941, and it has remained effective treatment for depression and schizophrenia.

ECT experienced its first widely criticized setback in Australia in early 1990s, following Chelmsford Royal Commission. Later in the decade successful attempts were made for ECT revival, by introducing modern techniques and, starting training programs for trainees and psychiatrists. In 2012 RANZCP, developed it as an Entrustable Professional Activity (EPA), outlining the proficiency in ECT practice required by trainee psychiatrists, before becoming eligible for Fellowship of the College. Despite its acknowledged utility, ECT remains controversial and stigmatized. Therefore Australia has developed more restrictive ECT legislation.

There are stringent rules about second or third opinion from psychiatrists for the choice of ECT and number of treatments, as well as seeking approval of Mental Health Review Tribunal, for involuntary patients. It is interesting to note that there has been significant decrease, in the number of compulsory ECT treatments and the number of patients, who received it since the change in the legislation.

Unfortunately the neuropsychological consequences of ECT can be distressing and incapacitating. Memory impairment is the major concern, which may or may not be reversible. Effects on anterograde memory, and in long-term autobiographical and impersonal memory, can be deleterious. With increasing number of ECTs, there is more likelihood of cognitive impairment, and post-ictal confusion, immediately after ECT, taking several days or weeks to resolve (Prudic J. et al 2008). These possible adverse effects should be discussed, with the patient and their family in balancing the decision to commence ECT. The other adverse effects include headache, muscle ache and dental damage. The adverse effects occur more frequently with bi-temporal for its direct stimulation of hippocampus, than with right unilateral ECT. It is of particular concern in the elderly, where they can develop delirium, during the course of the treatment.

In the recent years the use of ultra brief ECT has become more widely accepted, as it can preserve efficacy while reducing cognitive side effects. Ultra brief pulse width bi-frontal ECT is recommended, in preference to, bi-temporal ultra-brief ECT. The success of ECT depends on the seizures, within therapeutic range.

Male gender, older age, bi-temporal electrodes and anaesthetic drugs can increase seizure threshold. Some anaesthetic agents have anticonvulsant properties. All these factors should be considered to maximise ECT efficiency.

Following a course of ECT, relapse rates within 6 months have been shown to be over 50% despite maintenance psychotherapy. Therefore in some cases after the acute course is finished, periodic continuation up to 6 months and maintenance ECT (beyond 6 months) may be necessary

(Mood Disorder CPG). Ultra brief ECT can also be used effectively in continuation therapy.

Clinical practice guidelines for mood disorder published by RANZCP in 2020, recommends ECT followed by pharmacotherapy, as safe and highly effective treatment, for more severe forms of depression, where its antidepressant effect is found to be superior, to medication strategies.

Trans-cranial magnetic stimulation (TMS) repetitive trans-cranial magnetic stimulation is increasingly used, in clinical practice. It utilizes pulsed magnetic field, to stimulate and potentially alter brain activity. It is outpatient treatment without anaesthetic, 30 to 45 minute session, 5 days a week for 4 to 6 weeks. It has been the subject of intensive research, for well over 2 decades, and several meta-analysis have supported its antidepressant efficacy.

Deep brain stimulation (DBS): MRI based neuroimaging techniques have identified a range of brain regions, that are abnormally active in patients with depression: the target for implanting small series of stimulating electrodes, connected to pacemaker type pulse generator, placed below the clavicle in the chest. It is widely used in several neurological disorders. The evidence-based literature to support its use in psychiatric illnesses is, still waiting validation (Fitzgerald PB, 2015.).

Magnetic seizure therapy

It is similar to ECT where seizures are induced, by high intensity trans-cranial magnetic stimulation device. It awaits further research and evidence to recommend.

Trans-cranial direct current stimulation is application of weak electrical current to subtly modify brain activity. Research so far remains divided on its efficacy as an anti depressant.

TMS can be the option for treatment resistant patients, who fail to respond to multiple antidepressants and are not suitable for ECT.

Internet based interventions for depressive symptoms have demonstrated efficacy and can be considered as an initial intervention for mild depression. Mood-GYM (moodgym@anu.edu.au) is highly recommended CBT intervention to prevent and treat depression and associated anxiety.

Mostly, mood disorders can be managed as outpatients, but resistant depression or with suicide risk may need hospitalization

As much as it is evident, financial hardship is the strongest socioeconomic correlate of depressive episodes. Experience of deprivation is more relevant to mental health than other markers of social stresses. This is an intervention, to be initiated collectively by the government, via social and economic policies, in order to address inequalities, in living standards of its citizens.

St Johns Wort

Hypericum perforatum is a plant grown in Europe, West Asia and North Africa.

It is sold over the counter as St Johns wort in Australia, and is used to relieve mild to moderate symptoms of depression. The flowering tops of the plant have been used in Europe as an anti depressant agent since the Greek and Roman periods.

Although it is generally regarded as safe, there has been reported emergence of mania as well as serotonin syndrome, if taken with other antidepressants. In some countries it is a prescription drug, which has been recommended in Australia by the clinicians.

Minocycline: Inflammation has an established role in pathophysiology of major depressive disorders, and minocycline has been shown to modify immune inflammatory processes and also reduce oxidative stress and promote neuronal growth. Some studies have suggested its adjunctive role in the treatment of major depression (Dean OM, et al. 2017).

Dramatic slowdown of novel therapy development, over the past few years, has surged the trend towards repurposing drugs. Considered addictive in the past, like **ketamine**, **Magic mushroom** and **dexamphetamine** are getting a new lease of life, in a more respectable domain.

Stimulants

There are studies including, RCTs suggesting the role of CNS stimulants, like amphetamine, methylphenidate and modafinil, which have antidepressant effect on depressed patients. There have been reported significant benefits on intentional self-harm and suicidal attempts after initiating the stimulant (Rohde et al.2020). It is possible that by regulation of emotions and reducing symptoms of fatigue, stimulants may alleviate depression.

Bupropion though not a stimulant, has a few, amphetamine like characteristics making it a subject of addiction. Numerous patients, benefit by its inclusion in the treatment protocol, as an augmentation strategy for treatment resistant depression. Possibility of addiction must be considered, when a dopaminergic drug like Bupropion is administered for depression.

It was with great interest that I read an interesting report of, Faecal-microbiata transplants (FMT) for depression "Who, gives the capsule" published in the August 2019 edition of ANZJP. It was supported by ANZJP correspondence of June 2020, where, a 29 years old patient with long standing history of, bipolar 1 disorder and failure to respond to an exhaustive array of recommended treatments, finally responded to 9 FMTs over a period of 11 months. Within 6 months she was able to cease her heavy dosages of 3 mood stabilizers, and remained depression free, at her follow up nearly 2 years later. She was also able to shed the adverse effects of the medications, like losing 33 Kg of her body weight.

Diet and Body Mass Index

Immunity: the natural body defence mechanism is vital for physical and mental health. Oxidative stress has been widely implicated in a variety of disorders. Free radicals, in excess, inflict oxidative damage in lipids impacting on signal transmissions and brain function. Anti oxidants are, antidote to counteract oxidative stress. Individual oxidant level varies according to lifestyle, dietary and smoking habits. Deteriorating lifestyle factors such as excessive emotional stress, lack of exercise, alcohol and drug abuse induce free radical production in human brain.

Therefore attention must be focussed on simple discipline of healthy diet and body weight.

Diet quality is worse in people with anxiety and depressive disorders, and is linked to both chronicity and severity in dose response manner. It is plausible that diet quality and increased BMI, may influence the outcome of treatment.

A large multicentre Australian study supported the hypothesis, that a healthy, more anti-inflammatory diet and lower BMI, may enhance the efficacy of a combination of mitochondrial enhancing nutraceuticals in the treatment of bipolar disorder (Ashton M, et al. 2020).

Omega 3 fatty acid

With its anti-inflammatory potential, omega 3 fatty-acid may help alleviate milder cases of depression, when used as an adjunct to prescription medication. It can be given as dietary enhancement or supplementation.

Healthy life style cannot be overemphasized. Physical exercise, healthy diet pattern, non-smoking and adequate sleep have universally accepted benefit for depression. Nutrients consumed from diet, rather than supplements, are critical for brain function specially, the dietary quality like inclusion of zinc and folate for mood. Specific nutrients may target some of the key neurological pathways, to enhance response to antidepressants as well as, promoting neurogenesis.

As with any illness outcome, positive self-esteem is a reliable predictor of recovery. Older, married, socially involved and employed people with religious affiliation appear to have better self-esteem.

As in many other branches of medicine, in psychiatry treatments are not perfect but effective enough, to justify its judicious use.

I was relieved and delighted to see the commentary in the April 2020 issue of ANZJP by the editor Prof Malhi "No Bipolar 11-for me, or for you"

'It's all Bipolar, no subtype or kind. It is less confusing,

So, lets start using, simply bipolar,

And see what we find.'

I was always ill at ease with bipolar 1 and bipolar 11, being diagnosed with the intensity of symptoms and sharing the same treatment.

Placebo Although it may be an after-thought, it cannot be spared from any treatment plan or outcome. The placebo phenomenon has shown that the act of administering treatment regardless of its properties, can deliver health benefits. An individual's expectations, belief in its effectiveness, the therapeutic rituals and the psychosocial context of the treatment, can generate positive changes in the absence of pharmacological agents (Miller et al 2008).

Research shows that in the treatment of depression placebo used adjunctively with supportive care sessions can be just as effective as active medication (Leuchter et al 2014). Meta-analysis of clinical depression trials, report limited benefits of antidepressants, over placebo for people who are mildly or moderately depressed (Kirsch 2010). Placebo responses in clinical trials of anxiety disorder, can be up to 60% with long lasting and clinically relevant effects, observed in some trials (Schedlowski et al 2015).

The mind body dualism is very likely to play its role in positive thinking, stimulating the brain to release neurotransmitters and activating endogenous healing process. Natural history of resolution of symptoms with time cannot be underestimated.

Changes in depressive symptoms occur naturally without any treatment. Therefore placebo treatment also needs to be tested against no treatment controls.

Placebo can play a useful role in drug washout periods

Case Study

A single, 48 years old woman, with 2 teenage children who worked as a school counselor, wanted to see a female psychiatrist, therefore was referred to see me. She was ambitious, creative, independent and sometimes outspoken, even outrageous which resulted in her losing friends and perhaps her marriage. Generally she was high functioning though had periods of depression, when she became self critical and hopeless with uncaring of daily routines. There were long periods of remission when she did not see me for many months at a time.

Her periods of elated mood, confidence, accelerated drive and innovative ideas were most welcome in her life, when she became highly productive working on her projects and many extracurricular activities to the point of exhaustion, refusing to take her medication in case it reduced her energy, nor accepting the diagnosis of bipolar disorder. She lived through the phases of 'highs' and 'lows' from her early 20s and believed that it was her natural personality trying to compensate for her lows with highs. It was not till her children were born when she was confronted with organising her life to remain as a working mother. As much as she was admired for her efficiency and talents she started to get direct and indirect comments from her colleagues about her inconsistent behaviour. She was invariably late for her appointments either trying to fit me in her busy schedule or with lack of motivation to leave her home due to depression.

She took her children overseas for a month long holiday. Like many of her impulsive decisions she justified the expensive holiday on borrowed money, which was inappropriate under her prevailing circumstances. It took me a few years to convince her, of the need, to continue with maintenance medication, although she negotiated on the dosages, to keep it at low level. We agreed on regular follow up, and maintaining serum lithium levels, as well as accepting, mild deviation of her moods without altering her medication, which worked well for several years.

She remained generally well, with long periods of stability and acceptance of, minor mood variations. I considered our therapeutic relationship with open discussion about her illness, as the adjunctive factor for her recovery, as during my unavailability she found difficult to relate to another psychiatrist for the absence of mutually discussed management plan and her role in it.

Chronic fatigue Syndrome (CFS)

The undecided status of CFS still swings between general medicine and psychiatry. It is still debated if it can be distinguished from other medical and psychiatric diagnoses and similar other medically unexplained syndromes.

References

Akiscal HS, Pinto O 1999. The evolving bipolar spectrum: Prototype 1, II, III and IV, Psychiatric Clinics of North America.22: 517-534.

Ashton M, Dean OM, et al. Diet quality, dietary, inflammatory index and body mass index as predictors of response to adjunctive N-acetylcysteine and mitochondrial agents in adults with bipolar disorder: A sub-study of a randomised placebo-controlled trial. ANZJP. 2020 Vol 54 (2)159-172.

Bora E, Fernito A, et al 2012 Grey matter abnormalities in major Depressive Disorder: A meta-analysis of voxel based morphometry studies. Journal of Affective Disorders 139: 9-18.

Coupland C, Hill T, Morris R et al 2018. Antidepressant use and risk of adverse outcome in people aged 20-64 years: Cohort study using primary care database. BMC Medicine 16: 36.

Craddock N 2006 Genetics and mood disorders. Psychiatry, 5: 170-174.

Dean OM, Kanchanatawan B, et al. ANZJP 2017. Vol. 51(8) 829-840.

Deave T, Heron I, et al. The impact of maternal depression, in pregnancy, on early childhood development, International Journal of Obstetrics and Gynaecology 2008; 115: 1043-1051.

Dukart J, Regen F, et al. 2014 Electroconvulsive therapy induced brain plasticity determines therapeutic outcome in mood disorders. Proceedings of the National Academy of Sciences of USA 111: 1156-1161.

Fiedorowicz JG, Endicott J et al.2011. Sub threshold hypomanic symptoms in progression from unipolar major depression to bipolar disorder. American journal of psychiatry168: 40-48.

Fitzgerald PB, and Segrave R. 2015. Deep brain stimulation in mental health: Review of evidence for clinical efficacy. ANZJP 2015 49: 979-993.

Frey BN, Dias RS (2014) Sex hormones and biomarkers of neuro-protection and neuro-degeneration: Implications for female reproductive events in bipolar disorder. Bipolar Disorder 16: 48-57.

Geoffroy PA, Bellivier F, et al. 2016. ANZJP 2016 Vol 50(10) 1014-1017.

Gilligan J. Special Issue: Forensic psychotherapy: Applying psychoanalysis to the treatment of violent offenders. IJAPS2015;12 i-ii, 89-95.

Gitlin M et al.1995. Relapse, and impairment in bipolar disorder. American Journal of Psychiatry 152: 1635-1640.

Glahen DC, Curran JE, et al. 2012 High dimensional endo-phenotype ranking in the search of major depression risk genes. Biological Psychiatry 71: 6-14.

Hajek T, Weiner MW (2016) Neuro protective effects of lithium in human brain. Food-for-thought. Current Alzheimer research13: 862-872.

Haapakoski R, Mathieu et al. (2015) cumulative meta-analysis of interleukin-6 and 1 beta, tumour necrosis factor alpha and C-reactive protein in patients with major depressive disorder. Brain-Behaviour and immunity 49: 206-215.

Hannested J. DellaGioia N, et al. (2011) the effect of antidepressant medication treatment on serum levels of inflammatory cytokines; A meta-analysis. Neuro-psychopharmacology 36: 2452-2459.

Harris MG, Hobbs MJ, Burgess PM et al. 2015 Frequency and quality of mental health treatment for affective and anxiety disorders among Australian adults. Medical journal of Australia202: 184-189.

Horn R. 2006 Compliance, adherence and concordance: implications for asthma treatment. Chest 130: 56s-72s.

Javed Q, Dutta A. December, (2014) Third ventricle colloid cyst and organic hypomania, Progress in Neurology and Psychiatry.

Kirsch 2010 Review: Benefits of antidepressants over placebo limited except in very severe depression. Evidence-Based Mental Health. 13: 49.

Leuchter AF, Hunter AM, et al 2014. Role of pill taking: expectation and therapeutic alliance in the placebo response in clinical trials of major depression. British Journal of Psychiatry 205: 443-449.

Liu B, Wu Q, et al 2019 Lithium use and risk of fracture: A systematic review and meta-analysis of observational studies. Osteoporosis International 30: 257-266.

Lopresti AL, Hood ST, et al. (2013) A review of lifestyle factors that contribute to important pathways associated with major depression: Diet, sleep and exercise. Journal of Affective Disorders 148: 12-27.

Malhi GS, Adams D, et al.(2009) Clinical practice recommendations for bipolar disorder, Acta Psychiatrica Scandinevica 119: 27-46.

Malhi GS, Tanious M, et al. (2013) Potential mechanism of action of lithium in bipolar disorder: Current understanding. CNS Drugs 27:135-153.

Malhi GS, Fritz K, et al. Agitation for recognition by DSM-5 mixed features specifier signals fatigue. ANZJP, 2015, Vol. 49(6) 499-501.

McGovern A, Hamlin A. et al. A review of the antimicrobial side of antidepressants and its putative implications on the gut microbione, ANZJP 2019 Vol. 53(12) 1151-1166.

McMaster FP, Kusumakar V. 2004 Hippocampal volume in early onset depression. BMC Medicine 2:2.

Miller F G, Kaptchuk T J, et al. 2008 The power of context: Reconceptualising the placebo effect. Journal of Royal Society of Medicine 101: 222-225.

Moura C, Barnatsky S, et al. (2014) Antidepressant use and 10 years incident fracture risk: the population based Canadian Multicentre Osteoporosis Study. Osteoporosis International 25: 1473-1481.

Moya and Ferrer, (2016). Functional redundancy induced stability of gut micro bacteria subjected to disturbance, Trends in Microbiology 24; 402413.

Moylan S, Maes M, et al. (2013) The neuro progressive nature of major depressive disorder: Pathways to disease evolution and resistance and therapeutic implications Molecular Psychiatry 18: 595-606.

Opel N, Redlich R, et al. Hippocampal atrophy in major depression-a function of childhood maltreatment rather than diagnosis? Neuropsychopharmacology 2014 39: 2723-2731.

Muller N. COX-2 inhibitors Aspirin and Other Potential Anti-Inflammatory Treatments: for Psychiatric Disorders. Frontiers in Psychiatry 2019; 10: 375.

Paige E, Korda R, et al. Characteristics of antidepressant medication users in a cohort of mid-age and older Australians. ANZJP 2015. Vol 49 (3) 275-290.

Parker G Retrospective: Pursuing melancholia-The Australian contribution ANZJP 2017 Vol 51(1) 7-8.

Passos IC, Kapczinski F. Immune activation as a mediator of the gut brain axis in manic episodes. ANZJP, 2015 Correspondence Vol 49, no12.

Parker G. Pseudo-melancholia. Australasian Psychiatry, 2020 Vol 28(3). 339-341.

Perlis RH, Ostacher JK et al. Feb 2006.American Journal of Psychiatry Predictors of recurrence in bipolar disorder: primary outcome from systematic treatment enhancement program for bipolar disorder.

Pfaffenseller B, Fries GR, Wollenhaupt-Aguiar B, et al. 2013 Neuro-trophins, inflammation and oxidative stress as illness activity biomarker in bipolar disorder Expert Review of Neurotherapeutics, 13: 827-848.

Pfennig A, Leopold Karolina, et al. Longitudinal changes in the antecedent and early manifest course of bipolar disorder-A narrative review of prospective studies. ANZJP, 2017 Vol 51 No5 509-523.

Prudic J. Strategies to minimise cognitive side effects with ECT: aspects of ECT techniques. J ECT 2008; 24: 46-51.

Pruss H, Herken J 2017 Red flag: Clinical signs of identifying autoimmune encephalitis in psychiatric patients. Front Psychiatry 8: 25.

Rodriguez JM, Monsalves-Alvarez et al. (2016) Glucocorticoid resistance in chronic diseases. Steroids 115: 182-192.

Rohde C, Brink P, et al The use of stimulant in depression: Results from self controlled register study ANZJP 2020 Vol 54(8) 808-817.

Ruparelia N, Chai JT, et al. (2016) Inflammatory processes in cardiovascular disease: A route to targeted therapies. Nature Reviews Cardiology 14: 133-144.

Samame C, Martino DJ, et al. 2014 Longitudinal course of cognitive deficit in bipolar disorder: A meta-analytical study. Journal of Affective Disorders 164: 130-138.

Schedlowski M, Enck P, et al. 2015. Neuro-bio-behavioural mechanism of placebo and nocebo responses: Implications for clinical trials and clinical practice. Pharmacological reviews 67: 697-730.

Sebastian R, Hickie I. No gold medals: Assessing Australia's international mental health performance, Australasian Psychiatry, 2019 Vol 27 (1) 36-40.

Segal ZV, Williams JMG, et al. 2002 Mindfulness Based cognitive Therapy for Depression: A new approach, to preventing relapse. New York: Guildford.

Sidor MM, McQueen GM.2011 Antidepressant for acute treatment of bipolar depression: a systematic review and meta-analysis Journal of Clinical Psychiatry 72:156167.

Snyder HR 2013 Major depressive disorder is associated with broad impairment on neuropsychological measures of executive function: A meta-analysis and review. Psychological Bulletin139: 81-132.

Sowa-Kucma M, Styczen K, Siwek M, et al. 2018, Are there differences in lipid peroxidation and immune biomarkers between major depression and bipolar disorders? Effects of melancholia severity of illness episode number suicidal ideation prior suicide attempts and atypical depression. Progress in Neuro-Psycho-pharmacology and biological Psychiatry 81: 372-383.

STEP-BD (Systematic treatment enhancement program for bipolar disorder) American Journal of Psychiatry2006;163: 217-224.

Twomey C, O'Reilly G, et al 2014. A randomised controlled trial of the computerised CBT program, MoodGYM, for public mental health service users waiting for interventions. British Journal of Clinical Psychology 53: 433-504.

Yu C, Wang MYW, et al. Bradycardia and reduced exercise capacity associated with chronic normo-therapeutic lithium therapy ANZJP 2015 49, 7: 666-667.

Uvais NA, Kurian Jose. Third ventricle colloid cyst and chronic mania, ANZJP 2020 Volume 54 number 4, 439.

Veerman JL, Shrestha RN, et al. Depression prevention, labour force participation and income of older working age Australian: A micro-simulation economic analysis. ANZJP 2015 Vol 49(5) 430-436.

Wang T, Huang X, et al. Early-stage psychotherapy produces elevated frontal white matter integrity in adult major depressive disorders. PLoS One 2013; 8: e 63081.

Whiteford et al. Global burden of diseases attributable to mental and substance use disorder: Findings from the Global Burden of Diseases Study 2010. The Lancet 382: 1575-1586.

WHO Collaborating Centre for Drug Statistics Methodology, 2012.

Williams L J, Pascoe I, et al. Is there a nexus, between mental and bone health? ANZJP 2016 Vol 50 (9) 829-830.

Winter G, Hart RA et al 2018 Gut micro-biome and depression: What we know and what we need to know. Nature Reviews Neuroscience 29: 629-643.

Young J J, Bruno D, et al. (2014) A review of, the relationship between pro-inflammatory cytokines and major depressive disorder. Journal of Affective Disorders 169:15-20.

Zlatan Z, Weickert CS, et al. Neutrophil.-lymphocyte ratio-a simple, accessible measure of inflammation, morbidity and prognosis in psychiatric disorders? Australasian Psychiatry 2020, Vol 28 (4) 454-458.

ANXIETY DISORDERS

THE LONGITUDINAL COURSE of anxiety disorders is characterised as chronic, in almost 60% of cases after 2 years, and 20 to 60% cases after 12 years (Batelaan N, Et al 2014).

Generalised Anxiety Disorder (GAD): characterised by hyper-arousal, debilitating, chronic, excessive and uncontrollable worry, about a variety of topics, and anticipation of future threat. From evolutionary point of view, anxiety is adaptive, since it promotes survival by inciting the person to steer clear, of perilous places. Since 20th century, anxiety has been included in psychiatric classification. According to large population based surveys, well over 33% of population is affected by anxiety disorders during their lifetime. Substantial under-recognition and under-treatment of these disorders have been reported.

The prevalence of anxiety disorder is approximately twice as high in women than in men. Childhood sexual abuse, chronic stressors, genetic and neurobiological factors are possible causes of higher prevalence.

Anxiety disorders start in childhood, adolescence or early adulthood until they reach a peak in middle age, then tending to decrease with older age. fMRI studies of GAD have reported, hypo-function of prefrontal and anterior cingulate region.

Panic Disorder

Panic disorder is a relatively common psychiatric illness, leading to significant distress and disability. Major depression is a common comorbid condition.

It poses unique diagnostic challenge, due to substantial overlap with symptoms experienced in, myocardial infarction and cardiomyopathies.

About one third of patients with panic disorder continue to experience panic attacks and other symptoms, even after receiving first line treatment (Freire RC, et al. 2016).

Neuroimaging studies have consistently shown neural dysfunction in fear network, involving amygdala hypersensitivity, and lateral asymmetry in dorsolateral prefrontal cortex activity among patients with panic disorder, which reduces, after successful treatment with antidepressants or cognitive behavioural therapy (Presco J, et al. 2007).

The neuroanatomical hypothesis proposes, that brain stem and hypothalamus are responsible for the stress and panic responses; amygdala and hippocampus for fear anticipation and prefrontal cortex for phobic reaction and emotional dysregulation.

Case Study

A 28 years old highly intelligent mother of 3 children was referred for her excessive anxiety, which gradually worsened captivating her freedom, and undermining her role as a mother. She suffered from panic attacks leaving home, or talking to a stranger. Her panic finally led to agoraphobia, where she became increasingly confined to her home. She was an exceptionally caring mother, which justified her life style within her home: a cover up for her agoraphobia. She was creative and talented, designing and making, variety of crafts and needle work of professional level; all of which kept her happy; at home.

She was a champion swimmer as a child and was being trained professionally to national and international levels. Although it was at her parents' initiative, she started to enjoy it. About the age of 13 years she started to notice her coach's inappropriate interest in her body. She reported it to her mother who overlooked it, perhaps in the context of her expansive view of the future aspirations for her daughter. As it became more obvious making her uncomfortable, she started to miss her training, becoming sick or not trying her best. It immensely disappointed her mother. The training ended much to her relief. However she was left with unresolved anger not only towards the coach but also, against her mother who remained integral part of her life. The wedge between her mother and herself was never addressed and she felt that her father deliberately remained oblivious to her dilemma. She met her future husband about the age of 18 years, married him soon after and moved out.

Her panic symptoms started after the birth of her first child and steadily worsened. After taking over her management I hospitalised her, for trial of medications and for the hospital based Agoraphobia Program. She also attended several outpatient behavioural therapy programs conducted by multi-disciplinary team. Unfortunately nothing worked for her. Ultimately and reluctantly I relied on benzodiazepine and SSRI antidepressant. She was more productive in her home with well presented garden, taking care of her dogs and doing her craft work which, she started to sell at the local market accompanied by her husband. She enjoyed her culinary adventures. She had 2 more children. With support from her husband, who attended to all the business outside their home, she maintained a perfect home and the family life within the constraints of her illness. Unfortunately her relationship continued to deteriorate with her biological family specially, after her younger sister's husband tried to make advances towards her teenage daughters. She became estranged from her family, and chose not to attend the funeral, of her parents after their death.

My patient agreed to gradually reduce her benzodiazepine after 15 years, as it was becoming a concern for me. She successfully ceased it, after one year. Although she went out to the local club with her husband, did not venture out much more. Attending her daughter's wedding, preoccupied her for weeks before. She asked for her comforting dose of medication, which I am sure was only for its placebo effect.

She was generally contented with her life of the activities, she immensely enjoyed. We mutually agreed that the sense of her fulfillment was enough, not to subject her to the unrelenting trials of treatment to treat her agoraphobia or panic attacks, which she was able to easily avoid and coped well with it.

It was an important lesson for me that the treatment needs to be patient centered for returning them to a comfortable life and optimal functioning, which may not always be consistent with the guidelines of treatment and our expectations of 'normality'. Subjecting her to trials of treatment was unjustifiably traumatic, as she remained unwilling, undermining its efficacy.

Effective treatment options for panic disorder include psychotherapeutic measures such as cognitive behavioural therapy and pharmacotherapy. The latter includes both tricyclic antidepressants and selective serotonin reuptake inhibitors with benzodiazepine as adjunctive options.

Social Anxiety Disorder

Social Anxiety Disorder: a common and disabling disorder characterised by, excessive fear of negative evaluation and judgement, in social and performance situations, with blushing and submissiveness. It causes significant distress impacting on education, relationships, employment, and gaining independence due to avoidance and hyper-vigilance, leading to low self-image.

In Australia its reported prevalence is 8.4% (McEvoy PM, et al. 2011). It is the third most common psychiatric disorder, with poor rate of spontaneous remission. Older age, stable relationship and full time employment are some of the protective factors.

Functional neuroimaging studies have found increased limbic activation specially, in the amygdala and particularly in response to emotional stimuli of a social and self-critical situation. Oxytocin and testosterone, not only develop and execute our social and emotional behavior, but are also key players in adult neuroplasticity, playing a major role in social anxiety. (Viviani D, et al. 2011). The peptide and the steroid hormones have numerous anxiolytic and fear reducing actions, in the social domain, as well as powerful control over HPA function and activity, specially during stress.

Social anxiety typically precedes comorbid disorders. Agoraphobia is the highly comorbid disorder along with anxiety, depression, bulimia and substance abuse. Care must be taken in excluding transient anxiety, experienced normally during role transition, like starting school, a new job or having children.

It has mean onset from early to mid teens or even earlier, though seeking treatment is unusual, till it starts to impair social and occupational functions. Prevention and early intervention program must be directed towards this age. The treatment can be delayed due to fear of negative evaluation and uncertainty. One of the most extensively evaluated programs, 'Cool Little Kids' provides brief education for parents of inhibited preschool children. Online assessment and treatment services, such as Mind Spot Clinics: now offer with or without, face-to-face treatment. So these online treatments can now provide, complete service, including CBT with clinical outcomes, comparable to face-to-face treatments.

OBSESSIVE COMPULSIVE AND RELATED DISORDERS

FIRST PROPOSED BY Hollander in 1993, has been supported by wider community. A group of heterogeneous disorders increasingly described as having dimensional structure. They show high rates of co-morbidity with major depression and OCD with family history, suggesting genetic and aetiological association. It is conceptualised as ego dystonic anxiety, eliciting repetitive thoughts, images and urges; and anxiety alleviating compulsion of activity, causing significant disruption in life.

The group includes, obsessive compulsive disorder, body dysmorphic disorder (BDD), hoarding disorder, trichotillomania (hair pulling and excoriation (skin pulling) and hypochondriasis.

Trichotillomania

Trichotillomania is a relatively uncommon disorder usually commencing in early adolescence, with chronic course and rarely reported. Common in females: it is defined as body focused repetitive behaviour such as skin picking, hair pulling; usually of scalp, eyebrows and eyelids, and nail biting. By the definition of a ritualistic compulsive activity, with no purpose, it is classed as OCD related disorder. Detailed psychiatric evaluation to rule out any underlying pathology or consequential effect is recommended. Psychological and pharmacological interventions are most likely to be helpful (Sah DE, et al. 2008).

Obsessive-Compulsive Disorder

Obsessive Compulsive Disorder is characterised by recurring thoughts and beliefs, as well as physical and mental tasks performed repeatedly that are, difficult to resist.

Neurocognitive underpinning of OCD involves executive functions, like response inhibitions, planning, set shifting, and fluency, processing speed, attention, memory, and visual-spatial abilities. Lack of insight has been proposed as a significant impairment in recognising the absurdity, exaggeration and ego dystonic nature of the symptoms.

Most recent neurobiological studies now implicate prefrontal cortex (orbitofrontal and cingulate), basal ganglia and the thalamus to the pathogenesis of OCD (Pena-Garijo J, et al. 2010).

Classic psychoanalytic view hypothesises basic ambivalence in OCD to be caused by tyrannical superego, coupled with high level of aggression. Severe superego is thought to result from identification with critical and demanding significant other, while the high level of aggression are considered to be partly inborn and partly the manifestation of an excessive repression of anger (Kempke S, et al.2007).

Yale Brown Obsessive compulsive scale is the most well-known and used scale. It is composed of, a checklist with, some of the, most frequently reported OCD symptoms and of a ten item scale, to assess the severity of obsession and /or compulsion, according to their frequency, impairment, subjective discomfort, resistance and control over symptoms (Storch EA, et al. 2011).

Body Dysmorphic Disorder

Body dysmorphic disorder (BDD): defined as preoccupation with, some defect in physical appearance. The defect may be, slight physical anomaly, or non-existent, but the person's concern is excessive. It is globally more prevalent in women than men. With increased public attention on appearance and body weight endorsed by media, also increases anxiety, depression and low self-esteem (Pecorari G, et al. 2010).

BDD is relatively common in patients seeking cosmetic surgery. Some studies have found that preoccupation with nose, is the commonest complaint in BDD, which also has poor outcome. The prevalence of BDD traits among women seeking cosmetic rhinoplasty is 22% (Bellino S, et al. 2006).

Apart from anxiety and depression these patients may also share histrionic traits of seeking attention, narcissistic traits of their physical attractiveness and perfectionistic leanings of OCD with rigid and ritualistic behaviour.

Case Study

This patient was referred to see me by her family doctor, due to her perception of deformed nose, for which she was seeking cosmetic surgery. A 38 years old single woman was living with her parents, and worked in a well paying administrative position. She was older of two children. Although described as an emotionally sensitive child, she generally remembered her childhood as happy. There was significant family history of anxiety amongst the male members. Her mother's family took great deal of pride in their physical appearance. She herself was an attractive teenager, well disciplined, immaculate and compliant. Around the age of 16 years, she lost her grandmother to whom she was emotionally close, which was the start of her preoccupation with fitness and health. She spent significant amount of time in health maintenance activities with special attention to her body parts. In a distorted reflection of her face, walking through a shopping center she saw her deviated nasal septum, which initially concerned her, gradually expanding into preoccupation. She could not be convinced of its normal shape and variation. Her social life was affected as she stopped going out for possible embarrassment of being asked about her nose. She avoided people at work and started working in night shifts. Her anxiety and concern about her nose used up most of her energy, time and finances in searching for a remedy.

She wanted me to recommend her for rhinoplasty. With no insight, depressed mood, delusional belief of deformed nose and its obsessional preoccupation, she was at the verge of losing her job. Fortunately I was able to convince her of hospitalisation for intensive therapy which included, low dose antipsychotic, antidepressant and cognitive mediation as well as mindfulness therapy on alternate days. She was discharged after a month feeling more in control of her actions, improved insight, and acceptance of her body.

Treatment

Anxiety disorders are notoriously difficult to treat, as variety of genetic and environmental factors contribute to their development and severity.

Second generation antipsychotic drugs have also been widely used as adjunctive therapy to SSRI antidepressants: the first line of treatment guidelines recommendation, in patients with anxiety symptoms. These newer antipsychotic drugs have been shown to be effective in improving cognitive inflexibility, which involves dopaminergic dysfunction (Ducasse D, et al. 2014). Not all patients with OCD respond to medication.

Benzodiazepine anxiolytics have played a central role, in the pharmacological management of anxiety disorders for about 50 years. Although these remain effective in the short term, run the risk of tolerance and dependence with continuation.

Psychological Therapies

Cognitive behavioural therapy has been shown to be effective in wide variety of mental health disorders, and is used, to modify behaviour and self-control in, anxiety and related disorders. It is short term, skills-focused treatment, aimed at altering maladaptive emotional responses, by changing behaviour and cognition and providing better emotion regulation and awareness. The standard therapeutic approach is symptom provocation and response prevention, triggering and tolerating anxiety till it extinguishes. CBT alters neural circuitry underlying emotional processing and regulation.

Another simplified suggestion is distraction as sustained attention on daily activities, may reduce OCD symptoms.

Mindfulness therapy

Being mindful is an inherent human capacity, though not always easy to remain focused. It can improve with repeated activation, to bring the mind back to here and now. It is essential for any situation specially anxiety. Its increasing use in variety of illnesses along with meditation has, evolved over the past few decades as an influence of Eastern philosophy. Not only it plays significant role in self-control of mind and stress management, it has therapeutic effect on anxiety disorders and is a useful life skill to adapt. Both the patient and the therapist must aim to be mindfully engage. I have often heard patient dissatisfaction with an inattentive therapist, which undermines the trust and the outcome. Psychiatry largely relies on, verbal and nonverbal communication therefore it is vital, to stay empathically attuned and pay attention to big and small clues. Neurobiological and physiological impacts of relationships are bidirectional and positive connection is likely to benefit both the patient and the clinician, protecting from burnout and compassion fatigue.

Computerized, cognitive behavioural treatments programs, can significantly reduce, symptoms of anxiety.

Occupational Therapies

Remaining productive with goals and activities of interest as well as healthy lifestyle are vital in recovery. Vocational training along with all other treatment strategies will help, in gaining suitable employment, which remains a major issue, for any country. Mental disorders arise in context of, social and economic environment, which has direct relationship with employment. Analysis of cross sectional studies found that unemployment was associated with doubling of considerable psychological stress from 16% in employed population to 34% in unemployed population at least in the first 12 months (Paul K I 2009).

References

Batelaan N M, Rhebergen D, et al. 2014 Two-years course trajectories of anxiety disorder: Do DSM classification matter? The Journal of Clinical Psychiatry 75: 985-993.

Bellino S, Zizza M, et al. 2006 Dysmorphic concern symptoms and personality disorder: a clinical investigation in patients seeking cosmetic surgery. Psychiatric Research. 144 73-78.

Ducasse D, Boyer L, et al. 2014. D2 and D3 dopamine receptors affinity predicts effectiveness of anti psychotic drugs in obsessive-compulsive disorder: a meta-regression analysis. Psychopharmacology. 231:3765-3770.

Freire RC, Zugliani MM, Garcia RF et al. Treatment resistant panic disorder: a systematic review. Expert Opin Pharmacother.2016; 17: 159-168.

Kempke S, Luyten P 2007. Psychodynamic and cognitive behavioural approaches of obsessive-compulsive disorder: Is it time to work through our ambivalence? Bull. Menninger Clin. 71: (4), 291-311.

McEvoy PM, Grove R, et al. 20011 Epidemiology of anxiety disorders in Australian general population Findings of 2007 Australian National Survey of Mental Health and Wellbeing ANZJP 45:957-967.

Paul K I, Moser K. (2009) Unemployment impairs mental health: Meta-analysis. Journal of Vocational Behaviour 74: 264-282.

Pecorari G, Gramaglia C, et al. 2010. Self esteem and personality in subjects with and without body dysmorphic disorder traits, undergoing cosmetic rhinoplasty: Preliminary data. Journal of Plastic Reconstructive & Aesthetic surgery 63(3): 493-8.

Pena-Garijo J, Ruiperez-Rodriguez, et al. 2010. The neurobiology of obsessive-compulsive disorder: new findings from the functional magnetic resonance imaging (1) Rev. Neurol. 50: (8), 477-485.

Presco J, Zalesky R, Barnes M et al. The effect of repetitive trans-cranial magnetic-stimulation, add on serotonin reuptake inhibitors in patients with panic disorder: a randomised double blind sham controlled study. Neuro Endocrinol Lett 2007; 28: 33-38.

Sah DE, Koo J, et al. 2008 Trichotillomania. Dermatology and Therapy, 21:13-21).

Storch EA, Benito K, et al 2011 Assessment scale for obsessive-compulsive disorder. Neuropsychiatry 1: 243-250.

Viviani D, Charlet A, et al. Oxytocin selectively gates fear responses through distinct output from central amygdala. Science. 2011; 333(6038): 104-107.

POST-TRAUMATIC STRESS DISORDER (PTSD)

AT THE TIME of writing this book, there was, enough of national and global crises, for the forecasted potential increase in the diagnosis of PTSD, for many years to come. Disastrous bushfires, and pandemic Covid 19 will leave long-lasting memories of devastation. PTSD, as well as depression will follow the events and the impact of quarantine. We have experienced the sensationalised media coverage, igniting pre-disaster level of distress with cascade of negativity and emotional contagion. To minimise the post-traumatic stress, appropriate recommendations for required action were disseminated through media outlets

PTSD is a common and often a chronic mental health disorder, more often among emergency service workers and veterans, following an incident or cumulative occupational exposure, to potentially traumatic experiences. Inability to extinguish a conditioned fear is thought to be the core of PTSD.

In 2007 National Mental Health and Wellbeing Survey found that it was the most prevalent disorder in the country at 4.4%.

PTSD, is associated with, a number of physical co-morbidities, including gastrointestinal, hepatic and cardio-metabolic diseases, leading the calls for PTSD, to be recognised as a systemic disease (McFarlane AC, et al. 2017). People living with PTSD have low level of cardio-respiratory fitness, a strong independent predictor of cardiovascular morbidity, and mortality. The traditional risk factors like hypertension, smoking, diabetes and obesity are more prevalent in people with PTSD. Insomnia related symptoms are common, with suicidal thoughts and attempts. Suicide rates are 18% higher in transitioned Australian Defence Forces males, than civilian males. It has guarded prognosis.

The morbidity of depression and PTSD has similar impact in the terms of the function and impairment and yet, it has not received, the same intensity of, exploration.

PTSD is associated with dysfunction of immunological system and excess inflammation, which in turn is associated with significant cardiovascular health problems. Inflammatory changes in PTSD; are thought to be mediated by, a dysregulated HPA (hypothalamic pituitary adrenal) axis and epigenetic factor driving T-cells in to specific differentiation.

Chronic disorders like PTSD activate renin-angiotensin system leading to increased angiotensin synthesis, which promotes vasoconstriction, inflammation and fibrosis.

Burden of diseases arising from traumatic exposure is extensive, almost covering the entire psychiatric nosology. I started my training with dedicated Department of Veterans Affairs which has now merged with general psychiatry along with inclusion of all the stress related disorders like motor vehicle accidents, work related accidents, sexual assaults, domestic violence, burn injuries, and natural and man made disasters etc.

Royal Commission into Institutional Response to Sexual Abuse highlighted the trauma and the devastating life-long consequences of childhood sexual abuse.

The Military and Veterans' Mental Health Network was established in 2017 to assist the board of RANZCP to promote interest and expertise among psychiatrists, and trainees, in the mental health of military veterans and serving armed forces members.

The characteristic symptoms of PTSD include intrusive re-experiencing of the events, flashbacks or nightmares, avoidance of the reminders of the events, negative cognitive shift, and changes in arousal and reactivity. Symptoms lasting up to 4 weeks are classed as acute, and thereafter chronic, causing significant dysfunction or distress.

Longer-term subtle effects, can impact on psychological functioning, social and family cohesion, community structures and economies.

Some patients hear external, negative, persistent and controlling voices. The hypothesis put forward is: the disruption of cognitive domain that integrates consciousness, memory, identity or perception, as well as disruption of integrated auditory perception resulting in pseudo-hallucinations.

Post-traumatic intrusions may be misattributed by individuals to an external source and are subsequently experienced as hallucinations (Bentall RP, et al.2008).

The subdivision of sub-syndromal and complex PTSD with history of childhood abuse, need special attention due to mild to moderate symptoms, which can be overlooked.

Symptoms of insomnia, irritability, anxiety, startle response and social withdrawal can be misinterpreted, as normal reaction to abnormal events. However if these symptoms persist and concerns the person, it should be investigated, for possible early intervention. There is significant history of childhood sexual abuse in complex PTSD patients, making them more vulnerable to pseudo psychotic symptoms like hallucinations

There are reactive acute symptoms, which subside within short period. There can also be rapid escalation of problems, relating to substance abuse, self-harm and aggressive behaviour, mainly in younger people with poor coping skills and support. Older people with better premorbid resilience, and stable social network may present, much later after the crisis. They may present with cognitive or emotional symptoms-masking intrusive memories of the traumatic events.

There has been increasing recognition that the disaster itself is often the start of a complex series of events. The disruption distress, including not only the acute exposure, but also stressful life events, that may follow, including death or injury of family and friends, loss of housing, employment and income, damage to living environment (Forbes D, et al. 2015).

Risk factors for developing major depression and PTSD are: female gender, previous or family history of depression and history of previous experience of traumatic event and more stressful situations. Individual's emotional response during the disaster may play a critical role in development of depression and PTSD.

Nonetheless the good news from robust literature is that most people exposed to such trauma follow a resilient trajectory with relatively short-lived distress, which then settles (Bryant RA, et al. 2014) followed by recovery and stable mental health. However there is a significant minority who will remain chronically distressed or with delayed and worsening of symptoms.

Defence forces make up the single largest group of people, most likely to have the diagnosis of PTSD. Impact of military services on mental health and suicide, have been the focus of international research for sometime. There were 325 certified suicide deaths among serving or ex-serving (substantially higher) Australian Defence Force personnel, between 2001 and 2015. Transition from military to civilian life is identified as particularly stressful period. One of the most significant finding was that suicidality was associated with high loads of interpersonal and childhood trauma, childhood onset anxiety and high loads of adult trauma (Syed SA, et al. 2020b). Some studies suggest that childhood interpersonal trauma results in dysfunctional emotional regulation, which leads to suicidality in the context of challenging circumstances (Lemaigre C, et al 2019).

There are, other major life threatening events underlying PTSD. Many of these have been experienced around the world in the recent years. Apart from bushfires, floods, nuclear disasters and wars, earthquakes are regular occurrences in many countries as an endemic mishap. In September 2010, 7.1 magnitude, earthquake was centered in New Zealand at a depth of 11 km, destroying over 100,000 homes. The primary stress was immediate and obvious. The secondary stress, which affects mental and not physical health, seemed more severe, prolonged with ripple effects of disaster, and contributing to ongoing stress.

The more subtle effect of any disaster can impact on psychological function, social and family cohesion, community structure and economies.

Despite the range of psychophysiological and neurobiological abnormalities demonstrated in PTSD including inflammation, no evidence based specific therapy has been promoted. The extent of somatic symptoms such as chronic pain and comorbid psychological and physical disorders; need integrated focus of treatment and rehabilitation.

In treating PTSD patients, the concept of cultural competence consisting of core knowledge, skills and attitude is vital. Understanding the cultural context is fundamental to positive outcome. Treatment involved bio-psycho-social approach. The pharmacotherapy has generally been symptomatic.

Use of benzodiazepines for PTSD has been controversial. Although there is no evidence that benzodiazepines prevent or treat the core symptoms of PTSD; they do have a role to play, in alleviating the symptoms of anxiety, hyper-arousal and insomnia: often part of clinical presentation of PTSD (Roth LS. 2012). Tolerance to anxiolytic effects of benzodiazepines rarely develops in absence of substance use disorder, but tolerance to hypnotic effect is more common problem.

Both SSRI and SNRI are recommended by, the Department of Defence/Veterans Affairs. Overall treatment largely remains symptomatic, as no one drug works for all symptoms. Anxiolytic and antipsychotics are used to treat anxiety, anticonvulsants to treat impulsivity and emotional-lability and adrenergic agents like prazosin with caution, for reducing nightmares.

Rivastigmine an acetylcholinesterase-inhibitor approved for the treatment of dementia was reported, with promising success in an open trial of the treatment of chronic and severe PTSD (Murray A, et al. 2017).

Some PTSD patients with physical injuries like burn victims require multidisciplinary joint care, by medical, surgical and consultation liaison team.

Psychosocial support and treatment of PTSD is essential for better recovery.

Yoga: as an adjunct treatment cannot be underestimated as a potential treatment modality for PTSD.

Yoga has been used for thousands of years, to calm both mind and body reducing autonomic sympathetic activation, muscle tension and blood pressure. Yoga exerts positive effect upon neuroendocrine and hormonal function, decreases physical and emotional symptoms of distress, and enhances quality of life. Yoga has previously been acknowledged as a potentially beneficial strategy, to assist with the management of cognitive, emotional and physiological symptoms of PTSD.

The practice of Yoga is known to increase vagal tone, enhances GABA pathways in the brain, increases oxytocin and prolactin release, associated with positive emotions like safety, bonding and enhanced sense of wellbeing (van der Kolk, et al. 2014).

Neuro-feedback: As an adjunct to trauma informed therapy, it may help to remediate chronic PTSD related experiences. Evidence from several studies reports, improvement in sustained attention, cognitive control and working memory, as measured by, event related potentials. With lowering of higher level of physiological arousal and affect instability, the patient becomes more receptive to other forms of treatment (Othmer S, et al. 2009).

EMDR: Eye movement desensitisation and reprocessing therapy has shown promising response in PTSD. It addresses past present and future aspects of traumatic memory accessing emotional, physical and cognitive aspects of actual distress to traumatic event. This results in, changing the cognitive processing of memory, and cessation of trauma related stress, by using bilateral alternating stimulations and recall of traumatic memory. The bilateral alternating stimulations activate brain structures and its interconnectivity involved in fear extinction and extinction memory recall. (Fullana, et al. 2018). It also impacts on multisensory integration, memory formation and emotion processing.

Domestic Violence

Domestic Violence: In Australia male intimate partner violence has been found to be a leading contributor to death and illness for women aged between 15 and 44 years. A personal safety survey in 2013, of 1,494,000 Australian women, aged over 18 years revealed that 17% of all women had experienced sexual assault since the age of 15 years (Australian Bureau of Statistics 2013). At least one third of the reported homicide was, attributed to domestic violence.

Women who have experienced, violence during their pregnancy, have been studied and were found to have children with behavioural problems that can be measured up to the age of 4 years and beyond (Flach et al 2011). Chronic stress of domestic violence, which elevates cortisol, has long been known to cause anxiety and compromise higher cognitive functions.

A culprit of PTSD, domestic violence is increasingly recognised as widespread, and serious risk to mental health. Globally 1 in 3 women aged 15-44 years, suffer from domestic violence, responsible for 8% of burden of health. Majority of the victims are women, which is higher than smoking and hypertension.

There has been significant increase in domestic violence both in Australia and around the world as the direct result of Covid-19. Violence against women increases after major disasters, including fire, floods, hurricane or pandemic (Molyneaux 2020). Gender inequality impacts on women's safety during times of social unrest.

The succession of bushfires and Covid 19 in Australia has led to, increased periods of containment in the family household. In turn this has led to increased consumption of alcohol and drugs, loss of boundaries, powerlessness and lack of privacy. To the elevated level of domestic violence during this period, Australian Government has responded with substantial funding for the purpose.

It has come to the fore since it has become equated with punishable crime protecting the victim. As much as, one third of psychiatric patients, report it. One in 3 women and one in five men have experienced violence in intimate relationships (Oram S, et al. 2013).

The relationship between mental health issues and violence against women is complex. Women with diagnosed mental illness have increased vulnerability to physical and sexual violence.

Post traumatic stress disorder, anxiety and depression, are far more prevalent among the victims of domestic violence. Suicidal ideations are 4 times higher. On average one woman is killed every week in Australia by her current or ex-partner (White Ribbon Australia).

Case Study

This patient was referred to see me, by the social worker of the local hospital, where she was taken by her neighbour, following a fierce argument with her husband with threats of harm. She was living with her husband, their 3 years old son and her mother-in-law, since she married about 4 years ago. It was the second marriage for both which was, arranged overseas. She had a 10 years old daughter from her previous marriage, which also ended due to domestic violence, and she subsequently returned to live with her parents. Her parents responded to a matrimonial advertisement, of a man living in Australia seeking a bride.

She was a well-educated woman and did not want to remarry. However on her parents' insistence she agreed to meet her future husband. Her parents wanted to enquire more about this man but he wanted to marry within a week as he told them that he had business commitments to which her parents relented.

She left her daughter with her parents, and came to Australia with her new husband. She told me that soon after her arrival, she became aware of her husband's unscrupulous life style. She believed that his first marriage dissolved due to domestic violence. Nevertheless she decided to take the challenge, as she did not know anyone in the country, and could not bear the thought of disgracing her family overseas by her second marriage failure. She worked in the family business and had her son an year later. The verbal and then physical abuse steadily worsened, till she was, rescued by her neighbour. She finally separated, from her husband, with help of the Department of Community services (DOCS). Her husband subsequently hired a lawyer to claim the custody of their son, claiming that she was mentally ill. They obtained 2 psychiatric reports both condemning her as a parent with diagnosis of personality disorder and depression. DOCS then decided to get a report from me because of our shared cultural background.

Her husband and his family made an appointment to see me, which I cancelled and declined to see them. The court required me to present the report in person, which I did. The custody was awarded to her based on my report. I continued to see her for the next few months, when she made remarkable changes in her life displaying her strength and independence. She found a job, moved into an apartment, made some friends and bought a car. After nearly 2 years she returned to see me, to share her progress. She contacted her ex-husband's brother in Tasmania, who was a reasonable man, to connect her son to his father's family. All went well and her son visited his uncle and cousins in Tasmania, during school holidays. She got her daughter back from her parents who was now attending the local school. She finally got into shape, as a well placed, confident and independent single mother, with a few close friends and a social network. She told me that her parents were planning to visit her in a few months. She encouraged her son to visit his father.

Suicide

Suicide: remains leading cause of death in Australia, for people between 15 and 44 years of age. It claims lives of, 2800 Australians each year. The dynamic brain alterations in mental illness, is one of the leading causes of suicide. 25-30% of adults with diagnosis of bipolar disorder make at least one suicide attempt in their lifetime, and 8-19% of these patients die of suicide specially during depressive episode (Goldstein 2009).

Over the past 25 years there have been continuing efforts at national level, to minimize it, the last of which was 'Life in Mind' in 2019. In reviewing the impact of various interventions between 1991 and 2016 on suicide rates, the conclusion was that it has made no discernable difference

The National Prevention Strategy first introduced in 1999, formalized and coordinated suicide prevention activities, as well as provided for, greater funding and investment in suicide prevention research. While Australia observed decline in suicide rates following its introduction, this was principally related to efforts to reduce access to highly lethal means, such as firearms (Large MM, et al.2010).

Substantial number of suicide decedents, are shown to be in contact with a health care system during the month before their suicide. Therefore general practitioners, and other mental health professionals should be trained, for assessment and follow up with suicidal patients, with improved accessibility to psychological counseling and psychotherapy (WHO 2014).

The population of people who present to hospital with deliberate self-harm is one of the highest risk groups for subsequent suicide that any mental health service will encounter.

Although not entirely caused by mental illness/disorder, suicide has become a priority issue in psychiatry, for which a wider view is essential. It is complex interplay of cultural, bio-psychosocial factors, and it is argued, that it often results from, intense psychological pain, which becomes unbearable.

The impact of unemployment, being Indigenous, having sexual identity concerns, being in custody and experienced childhood abuse are the risk factors, which can be modifiable by lobbying for, broad social changes.

During our training, one of the important books recommended in the field of suicide, was of Emile Durkheim. His hypothesis of social, cultural and religious determinants of suicide, may also explain the poor results of various interventions, being offered without any sustainable impact, on the suicide rates. Therefore inclusion of philanthropic support has been a landmark, in expanding the meaning of suicide. Mental health services should also consider, social and cultural factors, in formulating suicide prevention strategies. Another point Durkheim has made was of social integration, which appears to be protective

(Durkheim E 2006). This may have been the reason for the decline in suicide rates after World-War 2, when there was greater integration of society, acknowledging publicly and privately, the impact of the losses.

Some people will always choose to exit life when confronted with a predicament. We must recognise that suicide is part of human condition.

In the ancient Greek city of Miletus (modern Turkey) the authorities were unable to stem a wave of suicide among young women. Eventually the decision was made to publicly display the naked bodies of women who had suicided. Suicides ceased (Beattie, 2015).

Young people account for one-third of nearly 8000 people across the globe who die by suicide each year. Therefore schools can offer an ideal opportunity for education and prevention of suicide, designed to reach the entire school population, which may be more acceptable by the students at awareness level (Wasserman D, et al.2015). Teaching young people to recognise warning signs of suicide, and empowering them to help their peers, capitalises on young people's preference for seeking help from their friends (Jorm AF, et al. 2007).

Teen Mental Health first aid program was developed in 2012 to meet the specific needs of upper high school years, reducing the help seeking barriers.

The program aims to increase mental health literacy, supportive behaviour towards peers with mental illness issues, reducing stigmatising attitude and help seeking from reliable and trusted adults (Hart LM, et al. 2018).

Role of medication cannot be overlooked as the cause of suicidal thoughts.

Isotretinoin (Roaccutane) hailed as a miracle drug for acne, was soon found to have the side effect of suicidal thoughts, and in some cases leading to suicide. Immune modulating agents have been associated with depression and suicidality. Natalizumab: a monoclonal antibody is used to slow the progress of relapsing and remitting multiple sclerosis. It has also been implicated in worsening of depression and suicidal thoughts (McCormack PL 2013).

Multiple sources of evidence suggest that brain derived neurotrophic factor (BDNF) is involved in the pathophysiology of suicide with its decreased plasma level, specially in pre-frontal and hippocampus, in post-mortem brains (Sher L 2011).

Testosterone is another neurobiological marker independent of BDNF, implicated in suicidal behaviour with significantly lower levels when compared with healthy control. Administration of testosterone is known to increase levels of BDNF (Carbone DL, et al. 2013).

Medicalization of every human emotion and professional intervention may not, necessarily help in preventing it. Suicide can occur in absence of any mental disorder as an escape from painful predicaments. WHO has recently declared the notion that only people with mental disorder completed suicide, to be a myth (WHO 2014).

Suicide, as the consequence of individual despair may be more related to individual personality and circumstances, like unemployment, family breakdown, loss of self-esteem and resources, which cannot be corrected by medications. There is well-recognised relationship between unemployment and suicide in nonclinical population. Even the impending threat of unemployment, within failing work places, may provoke a peak in distress and suicide, prior to the actual event. The risk of suicide may last well after the loss of employment.

Those who attempt suicide are not necessarily diminished in their capacity. It may be reflection of their own circumstances and their needs to be met, heard and understood (Janlowaski J, et al. 2013).

Personality factors are important in all the stress management initiatives including suicide.

In the end we must confess that we are unable to reliably predict suicide in an individual.

The impact of suicide on the psychiatrist is seldom discussed. Patient suicide is one of the most stressful professional events, experienced by psychiatrists or trainees. I can distinctly remember all the completed suicides of my or my colleagues' patients. It leaves you feeling sad, guilty, shocked and fearful with low mood. It may lead to acute stress disorder, impact on psychological well being, as well as on professional and personal life (Whitmore CA 2017).

Formal post vention guidelines and teaching about patient suicide and its effects could prepare psychiatry trainees to cope with this very stressful event.

Resilience

Resilience: can't be overemphasized in dealing with the stresses of life. In managing mental illnesses it is the integral part of response, remission and recovery. It is a skill, which confers adaptation, and is critical to the reduction of maladaptive behaviours, promotion of health and the prevention and treatment of mental and physical problems.

Resilience is described as positive emotions and optimism, ability to regulate emotions, cognitive flexibility, history of mastering challenges, commitment to a valued cause or purpose, capacity to extract meaning from adverse situations, high coping self efficacy, disciplined focus on skill development and altruism (Sher 2019). It is both innate trait such as personality and gene plasticity, and an attribute we develop from childhood to adolescence. I always believed that, an adverse situation: can either break you, or make you. Not everyone exposed to same situation will have the same outcome, or develop problems. Resilience is a multifaceted dynamic process involving acquisition and application of new skills.

Healthy life style, supportive environment, building positive emotions, security and self worth in daily life, are the prime ingredients of building resilience.

The continuing pandemic of Covid 19 is seen by resilient people as inspiring a master-class in adaptation. It has created new opportunities in the way we work and interact.

Resilient people actively create a world in which stressful situations are less likely to take place and adapt well in the face of stress and adversity.

Another group at the risk of suicide is veterans of combat and peacekeeping mission. Suicide rates were 13% higher for ex-servicemen when compared with, general male healthy population, according to Australian Institute of Health and welfare (2016).

The RANZCP clinical practice guidelines suggested that each deliberate self-harming patient requires assessment of modifiable risk factors for self-harm. It provides an opportunity for the assessment and treatment of underlying mental health problem. The period immediately following discharge is particularly important risk, for repeated self-harm and is at its height in the first 4 weeks after discharge.

Substance abuse, psychosis, mood and anxiety disorders, eating and personality disorders, medical conditions and relationships as well as social issues, must be explored for its impact on person's mental state. Living alone, high suicidal thoughts or plan, obsessional and anxious personality traits may need urgent intervention.

Therefore the current means of providing help may not be able to address all the underlying issues of nonmedical adversities of life.

Chronic suicidal thoughts may be amenable to cognitive behaviour therapy, which requires stretched out sessions. Unfortunately it is the acute suicidal thought, which need urgent intervention. There are not many options other than hospitalization for safety, which can give opportunity for treatment like supervised medication or ECT.

Ketamine

A non-competitive NMDA glutamate receptor antagonist has been mainly used for starting and maintaining anaesthesia and more recently as a recreational drug. It has also shown quick though short-term effect on lifting depressed mood. There are many studies of its beneficial effect on acute suicidal ideas. A systematic review and meta-analysis to determine the short and long term effectiveness of ketamine for suicidality, concluded that single dose of ketamine (0.5mg/kg) may have short-term benefit in the acute treatment of suicidal ideas. It also recommended one of the possible psychosocial interventions to maintain this effect (Witt, K, et al. 2020). Although there is considerable uncertainty about the use of ketamine, it may have a potential role as a therapeutic option in the clinical care of suicidal patients.

In another study potential efficacy of ketamine augmentation for treatment resistant depression showed encouraging results (Cusin c, et al 2017).

Assertive care after attempted suicide has been found most effective as a prevention strategy (Black Dog Institute).

There is extensive evidence to suggest that media reporting of suicide; can exert a contagious effect leading to copy-cat, imitating suicide acts specially if it is relating to a prominent person, with whom audience can identify, and providing explicit details about methods and location of death (Perkins J, et al 2018).

The media plays an important role in shaping attitudes and perceptions, of suicide. Reporting of suicide, illicit drug usage and similar anti mental health activities can have counter-intuitive effect making it more attractive and acceptable to vulnerable people.

On wider scale, media also makes huge public impact through silver screen. Many movies have been made to misrepresent both psychiatrists and psychiatry portraying them as non-scientific branch of medicine. "One Flew Over the Cuckoo's Nest" was one such movie based on Ken Kesey's novel of 1962 by the same name. The simplistic and inaccurate account of mental illnesses and its long outdated treatment that reinforces the fear of psychiatry in general public is: unfair representation of our helping profession. It is easy for media and vulnerable people to misinterpret and medicalise human problems without the endorsement, of professional bodies

Mind-frame a national media initiative: was established over 2 decades ago, as part of national strategy of the Department of Health and Ageing of Australian Government; for promoting responsible reporting of suicide and mental health in the media, which must portray suicide not as a way to solve personal problems. Responsible reporting minimizes potential harm, and enhances community understanding about suicide and mental illness.

Case Study

This man in his early fifties, who referred himself, can be easily described as worried well. He did not have any enduring symptom but just generally disillusioned with life. Coming from a modest family of a farming background, he completed his secondary schooling in the nearby town. Against the expectations of his family, he moved to Sydney where he completed his aeronautical engineering followed by MBA. He worked with Qantas for a few years before diverging in to a law degree. He befriended a, wealthy women and lived with her in an unfulfilling relationship for several years, before parting. He continued to see his 27 years old stepdaughter to whom he felt emotionally close. He often talked about her as their similarities in many ways specially, in their search for a fulfilling life. She travelled, worked overseas, tried illicit drugs and enjoyed some happy times with her family and friends though did not find the peace and contentment she was looking for. He wanted me to see her as he was starting to feel better more focused on his future plans, looking forward to positively integrating his life experiences, to find a meaning of life and self acceptance. There are some patients whose non-attendance is welcome and some you enjoy with a mutual sense of friendship within the therapy. He was the latter; who taught me some of the lessons of life. After some reluctance, his stepdaughter agreed to see me. I was pleased but not without some apprehension, in case I did not meet their expectations of changing her life. Nevertheless I looked forward to meeting her.

To my disappointment, an hour of her consultation time, remained vacant. My patient obviously was unaware of it. The next day I had an urgent call from this distraught man that his stepdaughter was missing since the previous evening. They went out for coffee a day earlier when she appeared pessimistic about her future, losing her motivation and drive, not sleeping or eating well and wanting to move out of her home implying that she had been a burden to her mother and sister.

The disappearance was reported to the police who rang him before his phone call to me.

The Gap is the ocean cliff on South Head peninsula in Eastern Sydney suburb of Watsons Bay, NSW Australia. Although a popular visitor destination, it has the infamy for suicides. About 50 people kill themselves each year by leaping off the cliff on the rocks or sea about 100 meters below.

The young woman apparently jumped off the cliff on the night of her disappearance when police search began. The next day a floating body was found a few km away at Circular Quay, close to where they met for the last time 2 days earlier for coffee. He was called to identify. He later described it as the worst day of his life blaming himself for not taking action before her disappearance.

References

Beattie D, Devitt P Suicide: A Modern Obsession. Dublin: Liberties Press. 2015.

Bentall R P and Fernyhough C. 2008. Social predictors of psychotic experiences: specificity and psychological mechanism. Schizophrenia Bulletin 34:10121020.

Bryant RA, Waters E, et al. 2014 Psychological outcome following the Victorian Black Saturday bushfire. ANZJP48: 634-643.

Black Dog Institute 2015 Implementation Plan for the Systems Approach to Suicide Prevention in NSW: Summary Paper. Sydney, NSW, Australia: Black Dog Institute. (https://nswmentalhealthcommission. com.au).

Carbone DL and Handa RJ 2013. Sex and stress hormone influences on the expression and activity of brain derived neurotrophic factor. Neuroscience 239: 295-303.

Cusin C, Lonescu DF, et al. Ketamine augmentation for outpatients with treatment resistant depression: Preliminary evidence for two-step intravenous dose escalation ANZJP 2017, Vol 51 (1) 55-64.

Durkheim E 2006 On Suicide Penguin Books.

Flach C, Lees M, et al. (2011) Antenatal domestic violence, Maternal mental health and subsequent child behaviour: A cohort study BJOG: An International Journal of Obstetrics and Gynaecology 118: 1383-1391.

Forbes D, Alkemade N, et al. 2015 Role of anger and ongoing stressors in mental health following a natural disaster. ANZJP 49:706-713

Fullana MA, AlbaJes-Eizagirre, et al. (2018) Fear extinction in human brain: A meta-analysis of fMRI studies in healthy participants. Neuroscience and Bio-behavioural Reviews 88 16-25.

GoldsteinTR (2009) Suicidality in paediatric bipolar disorder. Child and Adolescent Psychiatric Clinics of North America 18:339-352

Hart LM, Morgan JA, Rosetto A et al. Helping adolescents to better support their peers with mental health problems: A cluster randomised crossover trial of teen mental health first aid. ANZJP (2018) 52:638-651.

Janlowaski J and Compo-EngelsteinL (2013). Suicide in the context of terminal illness. The American Journal of Bioethics 13:13-14.

Jorm AF, Wright A. 2007. Beliefs of young people and their parents, about the effectiveness of intervention for mental disorder. ANZJP 41: 656-666.

Large MM, Nielssen O. (2010) Suicide in Australia: Meta analysis of rates and methods of suicide between 1988 and 2007 The MJA 192: 432-437.

Lemaigre C and Taylor 2019 Mediators of childhood trauma and suicidality in a cohort of socio-economically deprived Scottish men. Abuse and Neglect. 88: 159-170.

Mc CormackPL 2013 Natalizumab: A review of its use in in the management of relapsing and remitting multiple sclerosis. Drugs 73: 1463-1481.

McFarlane AC, Post-traumatic stress disorder is a systemic illness, not a mental disorder: is Cartesian dualism dead? Medical Journal of Australia 2017; 206: 251-257.

Molyneaux R, Gibbs L, Bryant RA, et al. (2020) Interpersonal violence and mental health outcomes following disaster. BJ Psych Open 6: el.

Murray A, Wallace D, et al. Revastigmine for treatment resistant PTSD ANZJP 2017, Vol 51. No 9.

Oram S, Travillion K et al. Systematic Review and meta-analysis of psychiatric disorder and perpetration of partner violence. Epidemiol Psych Sci 2013; 23: 361-376.

Othmer S and Othmer SF. Post traumatic stress disorder-Neurofeedback remedy. Biofeedback 200937: 24-31.

Perkins J, Blood RW et al 2018 Suicide and the News and Information Media: A Critical Review. Canberra ACT Commonwealth of Australia).

Roth LS. PTSD and benzodiazepine: A myth agreed upon Fed Pact 2012; 27: 12-21.

Sher L 2011. Brain derived neurotrophic factor and suicidal behaviour. Q JM: An International Journal of Medicine 104: 455-458.

Syed SA, Malhi G, et al. (2020b) Childhood trauma and Childhood Mental Disorder in Military and Employed Civilian Men Journal of Nervous and Mental Disease. 208:13-20.

van der Kolk BA, Stone L, et al. Yoga as an adjunct treatment for post-traumatic stress disorder: a randomised controlled trail. J Clin Psychiatry 2014; 75: 559-565.

Wasserman D, Hoven CW, Wasserman C, et al.2015 school based suicide prevention programs: SEYLE cluster-randomised controlled trials The Lancet 385: 1536-1544

White-Ribbon Australia. Domestic violence statistics https://www.whiteribbon.org.au/understand-domestic-violence/ facts-violence-women/ domestic –violence-statistics).

Whitmore CA, Cook J, et al. Supporting residents in the wake of patient suicide. Am J Psychiatry Resid J 2017; 12: 5-7.

Witt, K, et al. Ketamine for suicidal ideation in adults with psychiatric disorders: A systematic review and meta-analysis of treatment trials ANZJP 2020, Vol.54 (1) 29-45

World Health organisation 2014 Preventing Suicide: A Global imperative. Geneva: WHO

ALCOHOL AND OTHER ADDICTIONS

THE 2ND AUSTRALIAN survey of psychosis has revealed, the unremitting rates of smoking, alcohol related disorders and escalation of substance abuse among people with mental illness. The next survey in 2020 will shed light on the progress of improvement if any, in the lives of people who live with psychosis (Morgan VA, et al. 2012).

Clinicians in mainstream services are more experienced in recognising and responding to common physical complications of opioid and alcohol misuse disorder, and less skilled in screening, assessing and treating psychological harm, which can be more common and often more severe in methamphetamine users in comparison to other drug users (Duca Y 2019).

Opioids are one of the oldest drugs of abuse and carry, up to 60% risk of suicidal ideation (Oquendo 2018). The inhibitory impact of opioid substances on hypothalamic pituitary gonadal axis is well recognised. They hamper hypothalamic gonadotropin-releasing hormone resulting in testosterone reduction. It may lead to suicidal behaviour in opioid users. Testosterone deficiency leads to decreased libido and sexual activity, fatigue, erectile dysfunction, hot flushes, depressed mood, reduced memory and concentration, and insomnia, which are also the sign of opioid dependence.

Although relatively uncommon in Australia a patient with fentanyl addiction was admitted under my care which made me aware of its potential to become, a sought after drug for abuse. It is a potent and lethal synthetic opioid drug even in small quantities, which can cause life threatening respiratory depression. It is listed with strict restrictions of schedule 8 drugs, on the Pharmaceutical Benefit Scheme (PBS), approved for use in chronic non-malignant pain.

Amphetamine

Amphetamine and methamphetamine are potent and addictive synthetic stimulants, widely used internationally, favoured as drug of abuse, due to its psychoactive effects, resulting from its rapid transit of the blood-brain barrier.

Among certain subpopulations drug use is significantly higher in certain places like dance, music, nightclubs and music festivals. 642 surveyed attendees at an Australian music festival, 73.4% reported drug taking compared with 28.2% of the general young adult population, of which 59.8% admitted to using ecstasy (3,4 methylenedioxymethamphetamine MDMA) compared with 7%. 5 young Australians died at this festival. Evidence of danger associated with this behavior can be seen in the global statistics with 2.3% of Australian users seeking medical attention following MDMA use compared with global average of 1.0% (Alison Jones 2019).

It has been reported that President John F Kennedy received regular injections of methamphetamine combined with vitamins and hormones for his war injuries and to maintain his image of youthful vigour (Rasmussen 2008).

Resembling translucent stone or fragments of glass, methamphetamine was first synthesised in 1893 by Japanese scientist Nagayoshi, 6 years after the discovery of amphetamine. The mass production of the drug followed, the synthesis of its crystallised form in 1919 by Akira Ogata, and marketed for diet aid, somnolence and vitality (Panenka WJ 2013).

More than half of injecting amphetamine users, meet the criteria, of current or lifetime psychotic disorder (Hides L, 2015.) More than 16% of hospitalisations for psychosis in Australia, have comorbid amphetamine abuse.

Higher incidence of drug related hospitalisations alerted me, to the over diagnosis of Attention Deficit Hyperkinetic Disorder (ADHD), resulting in generous prescriptions of amphetamine.

I worked as a locum psychiatrist in a much-needed hospital, due to sudden departure of their long-term psychiatrist. To my surprise, majority of the patients came for the renewal of their dexamphetamine prescription, with a diagnosis of ADHD. As I was not comfortable in renewing the prescription without my diagnostic assessment of the patients, I suggested a new drug atmoxetine recently released in the market, instead. Obviously this was unacceptable. I was later informed that the black market price of "Speed", shot up in the town since my arrival. Walking in the hospital corridor one day, I met a past medical colleague, which surprised us both. He was quickly able to place me as the new hospital psychiatrist, subject of their AMA branch meeting discussion the previous night. The local general practitioners lodged a complaint that I was refusing to renew the prescriptions for amphetamine, unlike my predecessor who helped to keep the street cost of the drug at an affordable level by legal prescriptions. Obviously the family doctors were not comfortable in prescribing amphetamine.

In Tasmania, the per-capita prescription rate for alprazolam was, more than double, of the rate nationally (Galloway J. 2007).

With threats from the patients, hospital designated security guards for all my outpatient appointments.

Globally amphetamine use continues to rise. There is five-fold increase in amphetamine related psychosis admissions, strongly correlated to amphetamine availability. In Australia almost 1 in 10 people (9.1%) use methamphetamine. It is sold on the street under names of crystal meth, ice, speed, glass etc.

The formulation of crystal methamphetamine (ice) has come in the market of illicit drugs during the past few years. The typical users are mid to late teens, in their critical developmental period.

It is particularly neurotoxic in humans inducing psychotic symptoms, usually clinically indistinguishable from an acute psychotic episode in people with schizophrenia.

It can exacerbate or precipitate a more enduring psychotic disorder in susceptible individuals, as well as leading to symptoms of anxiety and mood disorders. The estimated prevalence of psychosis in amphetamine users is, 11 times higher than general population. Compared with other substances methamphetamine is highly neurotoxic. Its use can lead to long-term damage with concomitant deleterious effect on cognition, significant psychosocial impairment and poor developmental outcome.

Once amphetamine psychosis has developed psychotic symptoms can persists well beyond the acute intoxication and recur despite abstinence. Risk factors for developing amphetamine psychosis are younger age, using greater amount, premorbid schizotypal traits, major depression, alcohol dependence and antisocial personality disorder (Mcketin R, et al. 2006).

The presentation in the ED, of amphetamine intoxication can cause upheaval due to their agitation and aggression, using up more resources.

I was fortunate to be part of the research team of NISAD (National Institute of Schizophrenia And Related Disorders) over 25 years ago, where mismatched negativity (MMN) was one of significant project under the leadership of brilliant young scientist Prof Philip Ward. Although I was, not directly involved, but enough to understand, its relevance in schizophrenia research.

Mismatched negativity, an event related potential (ERP) is the neurophysiological marker of schizophrenia. It reflects the neural detection of mismatch between expected and deviant external stimuli. For instance bread and butter is expected and bread and apple are deviant. Another example is that the participant listens to a series of frequent standard tones that are randomly interrupted by infrequent deviant tones of different pitch and duration. People with schizophrenia show significantly reduced MMN response to deviant stimuli suggestive of a dysfunctional detection system at early pre-attentive stages. MMN is associated with illness duration in schizophrenia regardless of medication. It is thought to index neuro-pathological changes in the auditory cortex, which can contribute to cognitive deficits core of dysfunction seen in these individuals (Hermans DF, et al 2009).

The verbal learning and memory, working memory and executive functions, as well as cognitive flexibility are most characteristically impaired in schizophrenia.

Amphetamine psychosis shares with schizophrenia, the fundamental deficit in pre-attention auditory process and subsequent control processing as indexed by neurophysiological (MMN) and neuropsychological verbal, learning and memory. These markers may assist in identifying the amphetamine users who are likely to be at risk of developing schizophrenia.

Another interesting field of research to explore amphetamine related psychosis is the study of neurotransmitters such as glutamate. Hyper-dopaminergic state and NMDA receptor hypo-function, thought to be the core of schizophrenia. Healthy participants given the NMDA receptor antagonist ketamine demonstrate, reduced MMN with concomitant increase in psychotic symptoms. Thus the relationship between MMN and dopamine activity may be mediated via NMDA-glutamate function. Therefore it is likely that heavy use of amphetamine with genetically elevated dopamine may result in, excessive dopamine release and potential glutamate mediated toxicity (Lisman JE, et al.2008).

There are subsets of individuals who do not appear to develop psychotic symptoms with frequent use, and conversely some who experience chronic psychosis, following limited exposure to amphetamine (Akiyama K, et al. 2011).

Alcohol

Alcohol is civilisation's oldest and most widely employed tranquilizer but often defeats its own object by producing depression and addiction. It is puzzling to note that the hard attitude to cannabis is not, applied to alcohol, which is more dangerous. In 2014 Australia ranked 13th highest in terms of per capita alcohol consumption out of 43 countries surveyed by OECD (OECD. Statistics). National Survey of Mental Health and Wellbeing in 2007 indicated that 6.5% met life-time criteria for alcohol use disorder and 2.2 % met lifetime criteria for illicit drug use disorder. Problematic-alcohol and cannabis users represent 70% of all publicly funded treatment episodes in Australia (Australian Institute of Health and Welfare 2014).

Globally, substance use disorders were responsible for almost 20% of suicide related, disability adjusted life years in 2010, with 13.3% of this burden is attributable to alcohol use disorder alone (Ferrari A, et al. 2014).

As central nervous system depressant, alcohol intoxication can increase impulsiveness and psychological distress: known risk factors for suicidal behaviour. Alcohol dependence has been consistently identified as the second most common psychiatric diagnosis, behind depression for suicide. Relationship between alcohol, other drug use, and suicidal behaviour is robust.

Alcohol dependence can also impact on work and relationships, reducing social connections and support. Frontal executive dysfunctions, result in impaired problem solving ability and future orientation.

Young people account for 52% of all serious road injuries related to alcohol and 32 % of hospital admissions are for injuries from alcohol related violence (Kisley, S, et al. 2013).

Alcohol intoxication is the major contributor of road injuries, suicide, assaults and drowning. It is the greatest single problem; universities must address. Young people start using drugs and alcohol, anytime between 12 to 19 years. So school setting is the best place to start prevention and delaying use of alcohol. For this purpose **Climate School: Alcohol and Cannabis**; an internet-based interactive cartoon program was designed to inform harm minimisation (Botvin G J, et al. 2007). It is one of many strategies to prevent drug and alcohol misuse from early age.

For those who consumed more alcohol by volume in adolescence, the risk of substance use disorder and psychosocial impairment increased significantly. The risk of depression and anxiety increased in those who showed signs of alcohol dependence (Boden J 2020).

Alcohol consumption during pregnancy increases the risk of miscarriage, still-birth and premature delivery. It may be associated with alcohol related birth defects, and neurodevelopmental disorders.

Cannabis

Cannabis affects 13 million people worldwide, second highest global treatment burden for illicit substances (UNODC 2016). Australia leads the world in Cannabis abuse ahead of UK and US.

73% people with lifetime stimulant use disorder also had lifetime cannabis use disorder. Stimulants and cannabis can act synergistically, in worsening psychotic symptoms (Sara GE, et al. 2014).

Cannabis dependence causes impairment of mental health and general well being. Neuroanatomical alterations in the key areas of brain have been found, in neuroimaging studies (Lorenzetti V, et al 2019). The alteration was found dose dependent, heavier the use, more the changes, as compared to nonusers or recreational users.

The euphoric effects of Cannabis have been investigated for its utility in certain condition and it was found to be useful. Relaxation of Australian prescribing law in 2016 has led to its use as a medicinal cannabinoids.

There is evidence of its effective use in chronic pain, subjective muscle spasticity, short-term use in insomnia, and childhood epilepsy. Tetra hydro-cannabinol (THC) is also used for chemotherapy-induced nausea and vomiting, and HIV induced anorexia and weight loss.

According to 2016 National Drug Strategy Household Survey, more than 10% women of reproductive age had used cannabis, in the previous 12 months. Children exposed to cannabis in utero may have poor neurodevelopment, preterm birth, low birth weight, severe neonatal morbidity and death (Jaques et al (2014). The effect may be related to the carbon monoxide, generated by smoking cannabis (Newmeye MN, et al. 2017).

Synthetic cannabinoids have been available over the past 2 decades. Most have, greater agonist potency and affinity to cannabinoid receptors and, result in greater toxicity (Seely KA, et al. 2012).

Vaporised verses smoked cannabis is more severe with significantly higher paranoia ratings, cognitive impairment and greater neurotoxicity (Noble, et al 2019).

The outcome of Australian multisite treatment studies was, that there was significant reduction in criminal behaviour, psychopathology, IV related and physical health problems consistence with abstinence (Manning et al 2017). The recommendation for maintaining the recovery was continuation of engagement with support and rehabilitation beyond professional treatment.

Complementary-Medications

Disillusioned with the partial success of pharmacotherapy, increasing number of people, are turning to herbal medications reflecting on the growing market, for it. Subjects with psychiatric symptoms are more likely to use herbal medications than those without psychiatric symptoms (Eisenbergh 2001). With limited treatment options in traditional medicine and few side effects of herbal medication it is not surprising.

There has been reported importation of drugs, which may contain prohibited ingredients only available on prescription in Australia, and sold over the counter. It may have potential for toxicity and dependence.

It may escape the detection by the Australian Border Force Security for prohibited medicines specially containing opium. Having said that, there is rising global interest in, **Ayurvedic medicine**, which I guess is listed as complementary and alternative medicines in Australia. Ayurvedic treatment heavily relies on plants and herbs. Unfortunately there is paucity of literature available on the subject outside India. There is impressive list of plants with psychoactive properties, which can be used therapeutically and for its euphoric effect (Plants Affecting Human Mind: Jain).

Some of the commonly used herbal drugs are listed here.

Valerian

Valerian officinalis is a perennial plant found in North America, Europe and Asia. It has been used as sedative–hypnotic agent for over a thousand years. The enhancement of GABA transmission and the serotonergic effect via serotonin receptors 5A 5-HT5a are thought to be core mechanism of action (Dietz et al 2005).

Most reviews have reported Valerian as a safe herb with only adverse effect of daytime sedation. Despite inconclusive reports on the efficacy of Valerian, it appears to be a promising candidate, for the treatment of anxiety and insomnia (Mischoulon D, et al. 2004).

Passionflower

Passiflora incarnate has been used for anxiety and insomnia since ancient times. Its non-sedating anxiolytic effect has been proven in animal studies (Barbosa 2008). When compared with oxazepam for generalised anxiety disorder, it showed similar efficacy with subjective improvement, albeit with slower onset (Ngan, Conduit. 2011).

Chamomile

Matricaria recutita L is found in Europe and temperate regions of Asia. Dried flower heads of chamomile have long been used, as traditional herbal remedy to promote, relaxation and calmness, in the form of tea and aromatherapy. Neuro-endocrine modulation has been suggested as the mechanism of action (Awad et al 2007). Overall Chamomile is a safe herb with minimal side effects.

Ginkgo

Ginkgo biloba also known as, maidenhair tree, is a living fossil native to China. Ginkgo leaf extract, which is relatively safe, with few side effects, has long been used as a cognitive enhancer. It modulates cholinergic and monominergic pathways, and has antioxidant, anti platelet and GABAergic effect. It has been used with some success in patients with dementia and postmenopausal symptoms (Birks 2009).

Kava

Piper methysticum is widely used in Pacific Islands as a social and ceremonial tribal drink. It is known to reduce anxiety and insomnia with minimal side effects. However its hepatotoxicity neutralises any benefit (Teschke 2012). Kava is also known to modulate Cytochrome 450 enzyme, which can adversely impact on concomitant use of psychotropic medications

Prescribed Drugs: most frequently abused are: long list of psychotropic drugs specially, benzodiazepine. Launched in early 1960s it successfully replaced barbiturates at least for a decade when evidence for tolerance and dependence started to emerge, sometimes within a week. More recently irreversible deleterious effects on cognition with short acting or long-term use of benzodiazepines have been highlighted. Long-term use of hypnotics and benzodiazepine increases with age: highest among the elderly ranging from 7% to 43% (Donoghue J et al 2010).

It raises concerns about abuse and dependency. Sedation, poor physical functioning, depression and accidents are well known adverse effects, associated with excessive use of benzodiazepines.

Most psychotropic drugs are metabolised in the liver by enzymes of highly polymorphic CYP family. Genetic variation contributes to, drug metabolism and to total drug exposure, impacting on drug response, and liability to adverse effects. It has implications for poly-pharmacy, using several psychotropic drugs together.

Prescribed drugs have been used in injectable form, and special gel capsules specially, by opioid users, for its 'heroin like high'.

Smoking

One of the great quests of 20th century has been victory, over tobacco consumption especially in Australia. Unfortunately, this success is not shared by, the mentally ill people, who smoke twice as much as general population. 62% people living with schizophrenia smoke (de Leon et al.2005).

Nearly half of the smokers with mental illness have high or very high dependence on nicotine. With income less than half of the national average, nicotine absorbs most of it.

About one third of the adult smokers suffer from mental disorders like anxiety and affective illnesses. (Lawrence D, et al 2009).

Some researchers contend that smoking and psychotic illnesses share common etiological factors.

Long-term consequences of smoking are well recognised. Most of the smokers begin in their adolescence. Unfortunately, smoking is seldom addressed by, the health care providers, as in the light of their mental illness it is not considered, a predominant problem. They are rarely the subjects of, targeted antismoking strategies. Nevertheless tobacco legislation against smoking in public places appears to have made its mark, amongst psychiatric patients. Designated smoking areas in the hospital grounds, have further reinforced this message.

Quitting is challenging for a person with severe mental illness for various reasons including, the calming effect of nicotine. One of the options is switching to electronic cigarettes also known as vaporisers (vaping), which has become trendy among young people around the world. It delivers nicotine to which the smoker is addicted, without the product of combustion, which causes most of the adverse effects of smoking (Sharma R, et al. 2017). By augmenting several neurotransmitters, including dopamine, the nicotine of E-cigarettes, modestly improves attention, working memory and sensory gating. It may ameliorate sedation from the antipsychotic medication, and may counter some of the negative symptoms, improving social interactivity, albeit in short term. However, although E cigarettes may not be as harmful as nicotine smoking, it is still not safe. The Centers for

Disease Control and Prevention confirmed, 60 deaths, in patients with e-cigarettes or vaping product use, associated with lung injuries. E cigarettes can be used to quit smoking although in Australia it remains an illegal substance. However it is likely to be available in the near future for quit smoking program as a prescription drug dispensed by pharmacists.

There are, increasing number of young people, turning to the disposable, colourful and preloaded pods or sticks of E cigarettes because of its convenience, fruity flavour and nicotine like buzz, presuming that it is safer than cigarettes. Its relatively shorter introduction in the market since 2006, its long-term impact cannot be predicted. So the verdict on health risks is still out. With the controversial reports for and against the E-cigarettes, and to be on the safer side many countries have introduced either outright bans or severe restrictions on its availability.

In Australia E-cigarette use is trending upwards. National Drug Strategy Household Survey, reported rise across all age groups of people, who have ever used E cigarettes from 8.8% in 2016 to 11.3% in 2019. With WHO warning and Apple Corporation removing all E-cigarette related apps, Australia is also in the process of acting. It is likely to close off the loopholes of importing it, either online or as personal belonging

There still remains a place for behavioural counseling, support and nicotine replacement therapy. E cigarettes are not the best smoking cessation devices with its own potential for addiction.

As much as the nicotine may have calming effect on the mentally ill people, in some studies, early use before the age of 15 years may contribute to the risk of developing psychosis related outcomes by the age of 21 years (Rossler W, et al. 2015).

Risk of smoking in pregnant women with schizophrenia cannot be overemphasized. It increases the risk of low birth weight, preterm birth and perinatal death of the neonate.

Tobacco smoking reduces blood levels of many psychotropic drugs, by inducing cytochrome 450-enzyme CYP. 1A2 enzyme activity increase, up to 70% in heavy smokers, compared with non-smokers, from as few as 7 cigarettes a day (Faber MS 2004). Plasma levels of certain psychotropic drugs can rise significantly within days after quitting or reducing cigarette consumption.

Quitting can lead to significant improvement in mental and physical wellbeing and health and does not exacerbate pre-existing mental illness.

Behavioural addictions: are open to controversy and likely to be misused, as generally these are extension of leisure activities people engage in.

Gambling

Gambling a behavioural addiction is a widespread global and significant public health problem. Australians have highest rate of gambling losses in the world, at $1500 per gambling adult, per year, twice the rate of next gambling country, which is Singapore (Productivity Commission report).

Gambling provides 11% of state taxation revenue, the largest share of which comes from poker machines. Although only a small proportion of gambling is problematic, nearly 80% Australians reported some form of gambling.

Gambling is a common contributor to homelessness in elderly, in many Western countries, along with many other adverse consequences (Crane M, et al. 2005).

There is substantial evidence that problem-gambling can result in many adverse consequences including impaired physical and mental health, relationships and family dysfunction, financial problems and employment difficulties as well as legal issues (Productivity Commission 1999).

Gambling has also been associated with a range of co-morbid psychiatric conditions like drug and alcohol abuse, mood and anxiety disorders, and other impulse control disorders. There is some evidence that psychiatric comorbidity is associated with poor outcome and attrition rates (Hodgins 2010).

For those who do seek help, it is likely to be at the time of crisis relating to their gambling behaviour, which can offer an opportunity, to help the person overcome the addiction.

With the advent of technology, internet-gambling has become, a convenient mode of addiction. Both DSM and ICD have included it, in the list of addictions. Unhealthy behaviour and health problems are generally related to, poor control like immobilisation and inadequate sleep. In one study it was found, that internet-gambling, distracted over 75% of people involved, from work related tasks or other activities with negative consequences. 88% individual suffered from withdrawal symptoms within 3 days after stopping and 42% experienced more than 2 dimensions of impairment. This included impaired job performance, academic crisis and inadequate social interactions among others.

There is urgent need for coordinated approach involving mental health professionals, game developers and media to develop healthy approaches to gambling specially, internet-gaming, (Kuss DJ, et al. 2017a).

Internet addiction disorder

Defined as compulsive and pathological use of Internet.

While the use of Internet can be, problematic with its compulsive use and cyber-bullying, it is also a potential source of information, education and therapy.

Problematic computer use is, a growing worldwide social issue. It causes social, psychological, and neurological problems. China, where nearly 700 million people used smartphone, was the first country to recognise pathological internet-addiction as a clinical disorder, and there is international movement, to recognise Internet/Video Gaming Disorder. The proposed Facebook addiction disorder, and problematic smart phone use are, not far off. Facebook used by well over 2 billion individuals, has posted a warning about the psychological dangers, of passive scrolling which increases negative moods.

Brain changes, after social media use between the, ages of 6-18 years (NEJM 2016). It may be similar to those, in drug and alcohol use which triggers, deviant, dangerous and damaging behaviour, like cyber addiction (Mol Psychiatry 2016).

Children, who listen to music on the phone, play computer games, and watch videos, have delayed speech, dry eyes, short attention span, and loss of natural curiosity to learn.

Excessive Internet use affects cognitive and decision-making-processes, relationships, cyber sexual addiction, information overload, online gaming, and risky decision making by overlooking risks and hazards. Internet addiction is correlated with functional changes in the brain region involved in reward, conflict monitoring and cognitive control similar to substance addiction. With increased reward anticipation, and decreased realistic appraisal of the consequences, the risky decision making, may be a biological risk factor, for Internet addiction (Seok JW, et al 2015). Therefore it should not be seen as negative habit or behavioural problem, but clearly a pathological issue that involves reward psychology and related cognitive dysfunctions of ventro-lateral prefrontal cortex (Seok JW et al 2015).

Young adults use smartphones, to send mean numbers of 109.5 text messages, each day or approximately 3200 messages each month (Americans and text messaging). They receive 113 messages, and check their phones at least 60 times a day (Hartman, Sato. 45).

Case Study

17 years old teenager was referred to see me by his family doctor. He was spending 8-10 hours on his smartphone, a habit he developed over the past few years. He used to receive 200 messages a day. He took 3-4 minutes to respond to each message, amounting to about 10 hours a day, spent on texting and related activities. He admitted to losing control over his smartphone usage. It caused him finger pain, neck pain and sleep disturbance. His family time was drastically reduced and his academic work declined which triggered his referral to see me.

In Silicon Valley, famous for its digital technology, there is increasing trend to send their children, to non-techno school, due to the anticipated impact of social media on children's neurological development. Steve Jobs, who gave I-phone and I-pad to the world, kept his own children away from it. Bill gates did not avail his children with mobile phones, till the age of 14 years. Most of the high profile technology experts, limit their children's screen usage, be it television or computers.

References

Akiyama K, Sato A, et al. 2011 Chronic methamphetamine psychosis after long-term abstinence in Japanese incarcerated patients. The American Journal of addiction 20: 240-249.

Alison Jones and Jody Morgan Pill testing as harm reduction strategy: time to have the conversation MJA 211 (10) 18 November 2019

American and text messaging, http://www.pewinternet.org/09/11

Awad R, Levac D, et al. (2007), Effects of traditionally used anxiolytics botanicals, on enzymes of the gamma amino-butyric acid (GABA) system. Canadian Journal of Physiology and Pharmacology 85: 933-942.

Barbosa PR, Valassori SS, et-al. (2008), The aqueous extracts of Passiflora alata and Passiflora edulis reduce anxiety related behaviour without affecting memory process in rats. Journal of Medicinal Food 11: 282-288.

Birks J, Grimley. (2009), Ginkgo biloba for cognitive impairment and dementia. Cochrane Database of Systematic Reviews: CD 003 120.

Boden J Blair S, et al. 2020 Alcohol use in adolescents and adults psychopathology and social outcomes: Findings from 35-year cohort study ANZJP 2020 Vol 54 (9) 909-918.

Botvin G J and Griffith KW. 2007 School based program to prevent alcohol, nicotine and other drug use International Review of Psychiatry. 19: 607-615.

Crane M, Byrne K et al. The causes of homelessness in later life; findings from a 3-nation study. J Gerontol B Psychol Sci Soc Sci 2005;60: S152-S159.

de Leon and Diaz FJ 2005. A meta-analysis of world-wide studies demonstrates an association between schizophrenia and tobacco smoking behaviour. Schizophrenia Research 76: 135-157.

Dietz BM, Mahady GP et al. (2005) Valerian extract and valerinic acid are partial agonists of the 5-HT 5a receptor in vitro. Brain Research. Molecular Brain Research 138: 191-197.

Donoghue J and Lader M 2010 Usage of Benzodiazepine: A review. International Journal of psychiatry in Clinical Practice 14: 78-87.

Duca Y Aversa A, et-al. 2019 Substance abuse and male hypo-gonadism. Journal of Clinical Medicine 8: E 732.

Eisenberg DM, Captchuk TJ et al (2001) complementary and alternative medicines-an Annals series. Annals of Internal Medicine 135: 208.

Faber MS and Fuhr U. Time response of cytochrome P450 1A2 activity on cessation of heavy smoking. Clin Pharmacol Ther 2004; 76: 178-184.

Ferrari A, Norman R, et al.2014. The burden attributable to mental and substance use disorders as risk factors for suicide: Findings from Global Burden of Disease Study 2010.PLoS ONE 9: e91936.

Galloway J. New Restrictions, on Prescribing Alprazolam, Information circular for Pharmacies in Tasmania: Department of Health and Human Services, 2007.

Hartman, Sato. Cell phone use and grade point average among undergraduate university students. College Student Journal 45: 544-549.

Hermans DF, Ward PB, et al Amphetamine psychosis: a model for studying the onset and course of psychosis. MJA. Volume 190, Number 4. Feb-2009.

Hides L, McKetinR, Dawe S et al Primary and substance induced psychotic disorder in methamphetamine users. Psychiatry Research2015. 226(1): 91-96.

Hodgins DC, El-Guebaly (2010). The influence of substance dependence and mood disorder on outcome from pathological gambling: five years follow up. Journal of Gambling studies 26: 117-127.

Jaques et al (2014) Cannabis, the pregnant woman and her child: Weeding out the myth. Journal of Perinatology34: 417-424.

Kisley, S, Crowe E, et-al. A time series analysis of presentation to Queensland health facilities for alcohol related conditions, following the increase in 'alcopops' tax Australian Psychiatry 2013 Aug, Vol 21 No 4.

Kuss DJ, Griffith M, et al. 2017a. Chaos and confusion in DSM 5 diagnosis of internet-gaming-disorder: Issues, concerns and recommendations for clarity in the field. Journal of Behavioural Addictions 6: 103-109.

Lawrence D, Mitron F, Zubrick SR. Smoking and mental illness, results from population surveys in Australia and United States. BMC Public Health2009; 9:285.

Lisman JE, Coyle JT et al. circuit based framework for understanding neurotransmitter and risk gene interaction in schizophrenia. Trend Neuroscience 2008; 31: 234-242.

Lorenzetti V, Chye Y, Silva P et al 2019 Does regular cannabis use affect neuro-anatomy? An updated systematic review and meta-analysis of structural neuro-imaging studies. European Archives of Psychiatry and Clinical Neuroscience 269:59-71.

Manning V, Garfield JB, et al. Substance use outcome following treatment: Findings from Australian Patient Pathway Study. ANZJP 2017 Vol 5 (2) 177-189.

Mcketin R, McLaren J, et al. The prevalence of psychotic symptoms among methamphetamine users. Addiction 2006; 101: 1473-1478.

Mischoulon D. (2008) Herbal remedies for anxiety and insomnia: Kava and valerian. In: Mischoulon D and Rosenbaum JF (eds) Natural Medications for Psychiatric Disorders. Philadelphia Pennsylvania: Lippincott, Williams and Wilkins, pp. 119-139.

Mol Psychiatry 2016, 212:1781.

Morgan VA, Waterreus A, et al. 2012 People living with psychotic illness in 2010: The second Australian national survey of psychosis ANZJP 46: 735-752.

Newmeye MN, Swortwood et al. subjective and physiological effect, and expired carbon monoxide concentrations in frequent and occasional cannabis smokers following cannabis smoked, vaporized and oral cannabis administration. Drug Alcohol Depend 2017; 175: 67-76.

NEJM JW Psychiatry March 2016.

Ngan A, Conduit R (2011) A double blind, placebo controlled investigation of the effects of Passiflora incarnate (passionflower) herbal tea on subjective sleep quality. Phytotherapy Research 25: 1153-1159.

Noble MJ, Hedberg K, et-al. (2019) Acute cannabis toxicity. Clinical Toxicology. (Philadelphia, Pa) 57 (8) 735-742.

OECD. Statistics, http://stats.oecd.org/ Data Set Code=Health-Stat.

Panenka W J, Procyshyn R M, et-al. Methamphetamine use: a comprehensive review of molecular, preclinical and clinical findings.

Drug Alcohol Depend 2013; 129: 167-179.

Plants Affecting Human Mind (psychoactive plants) SK Jain Institute of Ethnobotany. Deep Publication.

Productivity Commission Gambling Enquiry Report. https://www.pc.gov.au/inquiries/ completed/ gambling-2010/report.

Rasmussen N. America's first amphetamine epidemic 1929-1971: a quantitative and qualitative retrospective with implications for the present. Am J Public Health 2008; 98:974-985.

Rossler W, Ajdacic-Gross V, et al. 2015. Subclinical psychosis syndromes in general population: Results from a large scale epidemiological survey among residents of the canton of Zurich, Switzerland. Epidemiology and Psychiatric Sciences 24: 69-77.

Sara GE, Malhi G, et al. Stimulants and other substance use disorder in schizophrenia: Prevalence, correlates and impacts in a population sample. ANZJP 2014 Vol 48(11) 1036-1047.

Seely KA, Lapoint J, et al. Spice drugs are more than harmless herbal blends: A review of pharmacology and toxicology of synthetic cannabinoids. Progr Neuro-psycho-pharmacol Biol Psychiatry 2012; 39: 234-243.

Seok J W, Lee KH, et al. (2015) Neural substrates of risky decision making in individuals with Internet addiction. ANZJP 49: 923-932

Sharma R, Castle D et al. Should we encourage smokers with severe mental illness to switch to electronic cigarettes? ANZJP 2017. 51 (7) 663-664.

Teschke R, Sarris I, et al. (2012) Kava hepatotoxicity in traditional and modern use: The presumed Pacific kava paradox hypothesis revisited. British Journal of Clinical Pharmacology 73: 170-174.

UN Office on Drugs and Crime (UNODC) 2016. Australia leads the world in Cannabis abuse ahead of UK and US.

EATING DISORDERS

EMOTIONS RELATED TO food, eating and body image are the core features of eating disorders. These are serious mental illnesses highly prevalent across the world, affecting about 8.4% of women and 2.2% of men with peak age of onset between 13 and 18 years. However all eating disorders can, and do arise at any age and in both males and females. Prognosis is guarded with mortality rate of around 2% to 5%. Psychiatric comorbidity like depression, anxiety, obsessive compulsive and personality disorders are common (Allison S, et al.2014).

Eating disorders, often comorbid with borderline personality disorder, generally start in mid adolescence. With considerable diagnostic instability and the course of illness, about 3/4th may improve, before entering adulthood.

Anorexia Nervosa

Anorexia nervosa is characterised by self imposed or maintained weight loss, dietary restraint and preoccupation with food, as well as overvaluation of body size and shape. It carries not only highest relapse rate, but also the highest death rate of any mental illness, where one in five deaths are by suicide. Suicide rate increases after 15 years of illness particularly in the context of, substance abuse and socioeconomic disadvantage (Russell J 2020).

Long-term recovery rate remains barely at 50%, despite boost in initiatives, in eating disorder research (A Phillipou et al. 2019). The bio-psychosocial model of illness is well accepted for causing, maintaining and compromising the treatment and recovery.

Negative self-concept leads to self-damaging behaviour. Starvation leads to blunting of affect, occasional brief episodes of elevated mood, loss of social and sexual drive, concrete thinking and preoccupation with food. Less prevalent are, potentially life threatening pancreatitis, as the result of malnutrition and superior mesenteric artery syndrome, which has clear association with anorexia nervosa.

Physical examination, is necessary part of assessment both to identify comorbidity and the consequences of starvation. It must include measurements of weight, height, blood pressure, pulse rate and calculation of BMI. Serum biochemistry as well as ECG if indicated should be arranged (Hay P, et al 2014).

Genetic studies have shown an overlap between schizophrenia, mood disorder and anorexia nervosa. In all eating disorders there is an increased genetic heritability and frequency of family history. Autistic social deficits and cognitive rigidity may be premorbid in anorexia nervosa but are exacerbated by weight loss.

Treatment of anorexia nervosa is challenging, as the patient is likely to experience strong feelings of anxiety to the extent of fear, when faced with food. It requires greater focus on bio-psycho-social model of illness. Re-feeding and nutritional rehabilitation should be the primary goal of the treatment.

Evidence for pharmacological treatment is weak. Pharmacotherapy is only effective to stimulate appetite, and treat comorbidity. Low dose antipsychotics like olanzapine may be useful in reducing anxiety and obsessive thinking though not without the risks of adverse effects.

Maintaining improved state of nourishment is another challenge. Outpatient treatment is the first line of treatment

Individual psychotherapies are limited. Maudsley family therapy with its limitations, and active involvement of the family, appears to have, some merit. Inpatient treatment may be necessary, if the physical health is compromised which may also face bed shortage. In New South

Wales day—hospital programs are being developed specially, in private hospitals, though not without limited availability and accessibility. Day hospitals have earned some credibility in treating eating disorders, even after their discharge.

The introduction in 2019 by the Federal Australian Government, of an extensive reimbursement program for the outpatient care of people with eating disorder, is timely and a major step forward. However realistic hopes and expectations must be maintained with harm-minimisation approach to medical complications, nutrition and weight control behaviour.

The effects of starvation are, likely to exacerbate psychological symptoms including depression and anxiety. These symptoms may be present before the onset of weight loss and may continue well after weight restoration and recovery, and must be assessed. Motivation to change remains strongest predictor of the treatment outcome. Patients are often unwilling to relinquish their symptoms or continue with behavioural changes.

Bulimia Nervosa

Bulimia nervosa: was, first described, by Gerald Russell in 1979 as part of impulse control problem. While anorexia has been given the priority as a most severe of all eating disorders, excessive and compulsive eating including bulimia is also coming to the forefront. Bulimia nervosa and binge eating are both defined as having regular and sustained binge eating episodes. People with bulimia also compensate for binge eating by irregular extreme weight control behaviour like, self-induced vomiting, diuretics and purgatives. So they are likely to be overweight or obese.

Obesity

Australia ranks fourth most **obese** nation of 31 countries reported by OECD, and eating disorders are on rise. It carries an increased risk for diabetes and cardiovascular diseases. It is a significant determinant of insulin resistance. Adipose tissues secrete adipo-cytokines a bioactive substance, which appears to mediate the development of coronary artery disease, through neuroendocrine dysregulation, and low-grade inflammation. Adiponectin a protective cytokines is low in obese people.

Physical examination is essential for comorbidity and obesity emergent health issues. Extracting true history and habits may be challenging as people with binge eating and bulimia are secretive and often feel guilty for their binging.

Treatment

Obesity is common in most of the psychiatric disorders, and is associated with poor course of illness and treatment outcome. Many psychotropic medications are associated with, weight gain and cardio-metabolic conditions.

The first line of treatment in adults with eating disorder is individual psychotherapy specially focussing on CBT. The latter can be provided in stand-alone therapy in guided self-help form. The other psychological therapies include interpersonal psychotherapy, dialectical behaviour therapy and mindfulness therapy.

Pharmacotherapy includes some evidence of tricyclic and high dose fluoxetine antidepressants in addition to anti epileptics like topiramate efficacy (Hay P et al 2014).

Bariatric surgery is becoming widely accepted as the most effective treatment for obesity. People seeking bariatric surgery have high rates of psychiatric and psychological problems with mood disorders as most common comorbidity. (Sarwer DB, et al. 2019).

Unfortunately surgery may not be the panacea for eating disorders, as the problem remains more deep-seated and emotional. Moreover weight regain occurs up to 27% in all bariatric surgery patients.

Body Mass Index

Body mass index (BMI) the ratio of weight to height has long been used to classify obesity for physical health. It is now being increasingly questioned, for not addressing the natural variation in people for their gender, height, age and tissue composition. As the new research emerges, there is more understanding of the fat which is desirable and which is not. Excessive visceral fat predisposes to the metabolic syndrome against peripheral fat, which is metabolically inert and stores toxic lipids thereby improving cardiovascular and metabolic health. Subcutaneous fat has been found to be associated with lower glucose and lipid levels, independent of abdominal fat (Porter SA, et al. 2009). Subcutaneous fat also provides crucial energy reserves during illness, thereby decreasing mortality. Loss of this subcutaneous fat from key areas of the body may increase the risk of diabetes and dyslipidaemia.

BMI can be deceptive, as people with normal range can have impaired metabolic profile and excessive visceral fat. Loss of skeletal muscle, as the result of ageing or inactivity can cause impaired insulin sensitivity, being the primary repository of glucose. As the muscle weighs more than fat, loss of muscle can give false sense of weight loss using BMI (Kaufmann C, et al. 2018).

Waist measurement captures the distribution of fat around the abdomen, which indicates the amount of visceral fat. The clinical recommendation is to keep waist circumference, below half of the height measurement, which is better predictor of type 2 diabetes and cardiovascular risks. Waist circumference divided by hip circumference appears to be more realistic. However these manual measurements leave room for error. There are other objective measures for accuracy used in research and specialist medical facilities like DEXA (dual energy X-ray absorptiometry) scan or magnetic resonance imaging. Ultrasonography is the tool of choice: more cost effective, less invasive which delineates visceral and subcutaneous fat thickness with acceptable precision (Stolk RP, et al. 2001). It is hoped that with advancing technology, causal role of obesity in health and illness will be precisely delineated to identify people at risk of developing diseases.

References

Allison S, Coppin B, et al. Fragmented Health care for anorexia nervosa. Australasian Psychiatry.2014; 22:306-307.

Kaufmann C, Agalawatta N, Malhi G, et al. Changing body mass index: The need for amore measured approach? ANZJP 2018, Vol 52 (8) 810-812.

Phillipou, A et al. A bio-psycho-social proposal to progress the field of Anorexia Nervosa. ANZJP 2019 Vol 53 (12) 1145-1147.

Porter SA, Massaro JM, etal. 2009. Abdominal subcutaneous adipose tissue: A protective fat depot? Diabetes Care 32: 1068-1075.

Russell J A bio-psychosocial proposal to progress in the field of anorexia nervosa. ANZJP 2020, Vol 54 (2) 202-207.

SarwerDB, Allison KC et al. psychopathology, disordered eating and impulsivity as predictors of outcomes of bariatric surgery. Surg Obes Relat Dis 2019; 15:650-655.

Stolk RP, Wink O et al. 2001 validity and reproducibility of ultrasonography for the measurement of intra abdominal adipose tissue. International Journal of Obesity 25(9): 1346-1351

CHILD AND ADOLESCENT PSYCHIATRY

"Ship is safe at harbour, but its not meant for it"

ACCORDING TO WORLD Health Organisation half of the mental illnesses begin before the age of 14 years, and 75% by mid twenties. Preventive intervention therefore, should target risk factors, in the earliest life stage.

The most significant and cherished, though challenging responsibility is to raise another human being and live our dreams, through them, creating yet another generation of hope.

Therefore the most important period of life, rightly acknowledged is childhood, as interplay of child's experiences and development, are important in determining the capacity of the grown up person they would be. Adult mental disorders emerge from multiple cumulative, and interactive effects of inherited genetic vulnerability, and negative exposures, that occur over the life course and, are often preceded by observable childhood psychopathology (Althoff RR, et al.2010). The interplay of nature and nurture is complex, and includes both the effect of maternal stress during pregnancy, as well as chromosomal, and epi-genetic effects. Therefore, early indicators of risk in childhood, that may be responsive to targeted interventions, in vulnerable children, may prevent adult mental disorders.

Australia is distinguished by its initiative: being the first country in 1998, to estimate the prevalence and burden of mental disorders in children and adolescents (National Survey of Mental Health and Wellbeing). It provided the basis for planning and development of child and adolescent mental health services in Australia. It was, followed by, 'Better Access', 'KidsMatter', 'MindMatters' and Headspace as well as online services such as youthbeyondblue, reachout and eheadspace. There has been significant investment, in mental health promotion and prevention, in a range of initiatives including school programs. The latest in the series is **"Be You"** a national program for mental health promotion and early intervention for children and adolescents. It was introduced in 2018 superseding previous programs, MindMatters and KidsMatter. The multimillion-dollar Australian National Mental Health in Education Initiative is freely available to all 24,000 early learning services, primary and secondary schools throughout Australia

The service use for mental health disorders appears to have, steadily increased thereafter.

The National Survey of Mental Health and Wellbeing revealed the highest prevalence of mental disorders, in the step and blended families or sole parents, their unemployed status and the rental family home. The parents and carers were not always aware, of the emotional problems, the children were suffering from (Lawrence. 2016).

The role of socio-demographic factors was not surprising, though the intriguing correlate: 'our young have better mental health, when their parents do not use English, as their main language'; certainly was.

The Australian population based studies, using the Longitudinal Study of Australian Children (LSAC), have estimated high prevalence of risk for mental disorder in 10,000 Australian children, aged 3 months to 13 years, using a wide array of indices spanning familial factors, and childhood antecedents (Guy S, et al. 2016). It is estimated that 13.6 % of 4 to 11 years old experience a diagnosable mental disorder in a 12 months period. Unfortunately the integrated services provided to the families and children, are grossly inadequate. Families therefore access support through a range of services including paediatric, nursing, NGOs and child protection services.

There are sensitive periods of brain development during the early years of life defined as antenatal period, to 5 years of age, when the key brain networks are established to support future social, cognitive and emotional capacities: foundation for functioning through the life course. The plasticity of the brain in these critical periods of development makes it highly sensitive to stress. Exposure to physical and psychological trauma can disrupt healthy development with cascading effect throughout the course of life. Childhood maltreatment negatively affects various domains of psychosocial development and is associated with emerging psychopathology in late childhood and adolescence extending to mental health problems in adulthood (Cicchetti D. 2016).

Attachment theory; provides a developmental framework of interpersonal experiences, that plays a role in regulating cognition, affect and interpersonal behaviour, and is associated with resilience, empathy, interpersonal functioning and psychological symptoms. Attachment bond and empathy start to develop in childhood. It is positively linked to securely attached children, compared to insecurely attached children (Nazarov A, et al. 2014).

Infant development is seen as occurring, in the context of caretaking relationships, and the quality of attachment experiences, as well as emotional interactions. Attachment trauma arises when the infant's biological propensity to attach to a caregiver is constantly thwarted (Liotti G. Training 2004).

Integrating neuroscience and attachment theory, allows for elaboration of the early development of affect regulation, and reflective functions, in the context of relationships, and relates to early traumatic experiences, to specific deficits, in the core psychological capacities of mental functioning

Individuals with high levels of anxious attachment needing approval from others, are likely to experience separation anxiety, and engage in an interpersonal style, generally marked by fixing attention, on distressing stimuli. Individuals with high level of avoidant attachment tend to feel uncomfortable with closeness to others and value their autonomy. They avoid distressing stimuli, and attachment related thoughts and feelings.

Anxious and specially avoidant adult attachments are more prevalent, in people with psychotic disorders.

Neurobiological research has identified a large number of key brain changes, including HPA axis and sympathetic and parasympathetic nervous system, potentially related to trauma with significant implications for mood and personality (Agorastos A, et al. 2018). There is increasing evidence that trauma plays an important role, in the aetiology of many psychiatric disorders.

Psychological effects of stress may also be influenced by, perinatal adverse event exposure during gestation and inherited susceptibility to a particular mental disorder.

Parental criminal offending, and exposure to family violence are, associated with later mental illness, as well as intergenerational translation of criminality, and victimization.

Internalizing vulnerabilities like emotions, fear and anxiety may be less detectable in class-rooms, against the externalizing risk factors, like responsibility, respect, aggression, hyperactivity, cognitive difficulties and inattention, which challenges, the discipline. These children were 4 to 6 times more likely to have been exposed to maltreatment, with greater risk for long-term adverse mental health and social outcomes (Green M, et al 2018-541).

Universal delivery of school based interventions to promote pro-social behaviour, and emotional regulation competencies, may be useful in preventing or mitigating a variety of adverse mental health, or other outcomes, in later life to which, the children in the risk category may be susceptible.

There has been wide recognition of discordant relationships and experiences within the family, with parents, peers, schools and teachers in personality development. Inadequate supervision and control, as well as parental overprotection, can undermine, raising a well functioning adult. There has been considerable progress in the field of child psychiatry, to highlight and address the risk factors, but to create a perfect world may never be possible. National Institute of Health and clinical excellence (NICE 2005) recommended first step in primary care of children, is to detect and act on psychosocial risks and child's environment.

The journey of a man begins with his/her entry into the world as an infant. For the fortunate ones, it is in the arms of a mother, which forms the foundation of all human relationships. Therefore there is emphasis on maternal bonding. A woman is more likely to suffer from mental illness following childbirth than any other time in her life. Around 15% women experience onset, relapse or exacerbation of, clinically diagnosed post-natal depression. The baby of a depressed or mentally ill mother is compromised in their bonding and early attachment impacting on life long ability to form trusting relationships. The concept of mother baby-unit is to build a life-long foundation, despite mother's illness. It not only provides opportunity to develop mother child relationship, but also builds up mother's confidence. There has been worldwide evidence of positive outcome of the mother baby dyad admission, to special clinics.

Most human behaviours and experiences occur outside conscious awareness. Traumatic events of childhood especially interpersonal, impact on cortical and subcortical system of brain, compromising its robust development and sequels. This understanding is vital in comprehensive evaluation of a dysfunction, in bio psychosocial framework. Fundamental social, emotional and physical development takes place in childhood, therefore early life experiences, are vital in shaping the human life trajectory, with special relevance to psychiatry. Both subjective and objective measures of neurobiological changes occurring in childhood confirm heightened reactions to daily stresses in adulthood who are also, frequent attenders of general practice (Glaser, et al 2006).

Negative long-term outcome for toddlers and Pre School aged children displaying early behavioural problems are known to be far reaching.

Major risk factors for physical illnesses are well publicised and routinely followed up, the risk factors however for mental disorders are difficult to publicise or modify. With challenges in finding cure for most illnesses, prevention is becoming an important part of heath care, which includes reducing the risk, and enhancing protective factors.

Socioeconomic environment, adverse childhood experiences, disrupted family, educational level; parental control, child maltreatment, parental mental illnesses, drug and alcohol use, interpersonal as well as community violence and bullying are some of the risk factors for children. Well-nourished child with adequate sleep may be the starting point. Sleeping less than 8 hours per night, have increased risk of a broad range of health and other problems, including poor academic performance, obesity and increased risk of suicide (Lui X. 2004).

Improving parental skills and maternal health, including knowledge, skills and diligence is, the ethical obligation for better outcome. The emerging success of mindfulness-based research has expanded in the arena of parenting as well. Mindful parenting includes listening, nonjudgmental acceptance, compassion, self-regulation, and emotional awareness. The strength of mindful-parenting is its ability to reduce parental anger, stress and reactivity

To involve the children in parental mental illness or not is no longer a question, due to its impact on all family members. It may give the child an important role in the family, being valued, to share the responsibility. The positive experience will be, an opportunity to strengthen and build on their capacity to manage, and make sense of their home situation, and their parent's illness. If needed it can be part of family therapy.

Case Study The leaving of Liverpool

"The best way to make children good is to make them happy"
-Oscar Wilde, author and poet

In 1992 I was compelled to see, a highly recommended powerful and emotional ABC produced movie "The Leaving of Liverpool". I already met at least 4 of the survivors, of the huge child migration scheme of British Government in the post war 1950s, to add to the educated white population, of the far-flung corners of their Empire like Australia, New Zealand and Canada; on which the movie was based. Unbeknown to an average Australian the movie generated huge public interest both in UK and Australia.

My contacts came from a little known town in Central Western NSW in Australia, which became notorious for opening up yet another orphanage, to ruthlessly betray the children, who arrived from already brutalised and dehumanising treatment of the so called 'caring' religious institution in Liverpool UK.

I saw this patient for many years, a handsome, hardworking intelligent man with affable personality, I couldn't help liking. He had faint memories of the last visit of his mother, about the age of 8 years when he, along with his brother and their sister were promised by their mother to return home (near London) very soon. Each day in the orphanage still in UK as he slogged with the orders given by the nuns: his carers, he was comforted by hearing the words of his mother in his mind, to return, who never came as she promised. Instead the news came that he along with other children will be moving overseas for an adventure trip. The news got him worried in case mum turned up. But like it or not he was shipped out on months long treacherous journey to Australia. He panicked in the foreign land so far away from the images of his mother. On arrival the children were placed, without any consideration of the relationships and strong mutual bond, they formed with one another on their journey to their new home: the only security they were hanging on to, in the alien world. Years later he was told by a friend to check out in another hostel and another school down the road as a boy looked very much like him. He rushed and sure it was, his long lost brother. They could not find the whereabouts of their sister, whom they last saw on the ship.

My patient on one side was a charming, handsome and highly Intelligent, 10 years old boy, who had dreams of climbing the Mt Everest, and returning back to his mother, pledging to change the world, so that no child will ever live through his experiences. On the other side however in his real life, he lived in the gruesome abuse of cold water in the freezing winter of his new home, and working on the farm before and after school, with the harsh discipline and penalties from the heartless nuns. The close bond between the children, and the boundless human resilience was their only strength.

He finally was released at the age of 18yrs, to fend for himself. Not surprising, he found the transient joys of illicit drugs and alcohol, before expanding on his new adventures of life. The journey from here took him further and further, from his childhood dreams. I saw him in his early 40s. He married a stunning beauty from NZ, with similar background. They struggled together through recurring turbulence, and raised 2 beautiful daughters, whom they loved dearly. He later separated from his wife, though never stopped loving her. He was shattered, when he lost her a year later from cancer. He never recovered from it. Both of his daughters married, with his deadly fear of yet another generation of dysfunctional family

I often thought of his fate. The journey and the destination could have been vastly different, had he been raised differently. Not knowing the circumstances of his entry into the orphanage, and picking up on some of his natural assets, my guess was that he had healthy genetic endowment. It was the extreme form of childhood abuse, which changed his path and stole his dreams of, climbing the Mt Everest.

He left me with profound feelings of sadness, guilt and remorse, on behalf of my fellow human-beings, from another era, and more so with the sense of gratitude to him for trusting me.

My other three ex residents of the same children's home were not dissimilar, who suffered from lifelong flashbacks, panic attacks, nightmares, black depression and attempted suicides. Most of the children exported from Liverpool UK, for a 'better life' in Australia, received lifelong ongoing psychiatric care, albeit there were a few, who rose to prominence, due to their successful career, though on the personal level, none could forget the torture, in the hands of their carer.

This I considered one of the worst mistakes almost to criminal level, committed by the regime of the time in managing other people's children

"There can be no keener revelation of a society's soul than the way in which it treats its children" Nelson Mandela.

Child maltreatment is a serious global issue not only in low-income countries but in affluent societies as well. It requires stern action at international and national levels, involving health professionals, law, makers and enforcers.

The profound impact of childhood trauma is, not only limited to adverse emotional and social consequences: it irreversibly impairs the integrity of brain. Grey matter, hippocampal and amygdala volume reduction and cortical thinning resulting from childhood trauma are linked with increased risk of developing psychosis and poor functioning (Aas M, et al. 2012). It has epigenetic effects impacting on intergenerational risks of life long adversities.

Childhood trauma not only destroys the child in their adulthood but also weakens, the potential of the country in its future progress.

The National Mental Health Benchmarking (child and adolescent) Project was conducted between 2005 and 2008, as one of the National Mental Health Strategy's initiative, to improve service quality. It brought together 23 mental health organisations from across Australia, to attend series of forums, at which the organisations could benchmark themselves, against each other. It has potential to identify key performance indicators, as well as highlight intra and inter organisational performance.

Self-Harm

Self-Harm: Deliberate self-harm is, one of the highest risk groups for, subsequent suicide that, any mental health service will encounter.

Non-fatal suicidal thoughts and behaviours are common, need close follow-up, as moderate proportion of people about one in five, will progress to suicide attempt within 12 months, and a small proportion will succumb, to death (Bostwick 2016). However, most of the self-harming people, will not die by suicide, but from wide range of other related causes. Self-harming behaviours have significant public health implications in their own right.

Relatively rare before, self-harm has steadily become not so uncommon over the past 2 decades, at least in my experience. Mental disorders make a major contribution to adolescent health, and so does the desire to hurt oneself.

Deliberate self-harm makes significant contribution, to the burden of disease and is, the second leading cause of death among 15 to 24 years old Australians (Mathews R, et al. 2011) In Australia 1 in 10 teenagers have self-harmed, 1 in 13 have contemplated suicide, 1 in 20 have made a plan and 1 in 40 have attempted suicide (Lawrence D, et al 2015). The average age of self-harm is 12-14 years though there is reported one third who may initiate it, in late adolescence or mid 20s. For most adolescents self-harm resolves spontaneously, though for some it may continue well into their adulthood particularly for females (Stanford S, 2017).

Self-harming people may also have a range of health risk behaviours, like smoking, drug and alcohol misuse and other antisocial behaviours, which carry profound lifelong health and social consequences. In one study the predictors of self-harm included maternal depression, affective dys-regulation and homosexual orientation.

Deliberate self-harm is markedly increased in borderline personality disorders, with prevalence of 75% compared to up to 20% in general psychiatric population.

There is no evidence of efficacy of pharmacotherapy, which should only be prescribed if otherwise indicated.

A type of psycho-dynamically informed treatment, mentalisation based therapy and dialectical based therapies, have shown promise in reducing deliberate self-harm and suicidal behaviour. It uses empathy, encouragement and validation of emotional stress, together with determined focus on the mental-state representation that, contributes to stress, by reflecting on their, as well as other's mind (Bateman A, et al 2009). Generally the treatment aim should be multifaceted. A thorough assessment and formulation of premorbid difficulties to inform multidisciplinary treatment planning is a good start. Possibility of psychotic illness in major self-mutilation must be excluded.

UN agency states that countries can only harness the economic potential of the youth bulge, if they are able to provide good health, quality education, and suitable employment, to its entire population.

Suicide

He was a 14 years old boy from my social network, found by the school cleaner, hanging from the ceiling. It deeply hit home: the impact was incomprehensible. Older of 2 children, he recently moved to this prestigious boys school, a good student with attractive personality surprised everyone as there was no sign of warning. The school organised a heart-wrenching-farewell, where teachers and the students cried with the family: unforgettable life-event, for anyone.

Suicide remains the leading cause of death in youth aged 15 to 24 years, and for every young person that takes their own life, there are up to 200 suicide attempts. The reasons behind are likely to be school related, like bullying and the performance pressures, which involves the role of the school. Psycho-education should be part of the curriculum for the awareness and knowledge of mental illness and suicide risks. Student suicide must be handled with great deal of sensitivity and care to avoid distress and trauma to the teachers and students. Cluster suicides are more common in adolescents than adults.

Bullying

Bullying is an international public health problem, ranging between 10%-30% (Analitis F, et al.2009). It is defined as intentional and repeated harm, of a less powerful individual.

One in 4 Australian school children aged between 8 and 14 years frequently experience bullying-victimisation, which can lead to higher risk of self-harm, suicidal behaviour, and substance abuse. Suicide is one of the most serious mental health problems, related to school bullying, and has generated much attention. It can be in the form of physical threat, harm, name calling, teasing, spreading rumours and excluding from a group, as well as cyber-bullying. Those bullied, demonstrated depressive symptoms such as poor social and emotional adjustment, greater difficulty making friends, poor relationship with classmates and greater loneliness. Bullying victimisation, as a stress factor or trauma, may also contribute to the aggravation of psychotic symptoms, or accelerate the transition to psychotic disorders, in vulnerable adolescents (van Dam DS, et al 2012).

With the increased use of technology, there has been surge of cyber bullying over the last decade among both primary and secondary students. Text messaging, social networking and photo sharing applications stakes for creating electronic, immediately and widely distributable messages and images. Cyber bullying violates many social norms and potentially includes criminal behaviour such as harassment, stalking, pornography and incitement of individuals to harm or kill themselves (Scott J et al. 2014).

Although the school may not be the primary platform, cyber bullying is often linked to peer relationships.

Both victims and the bully-victims are at the highest risk of, adverse mental health outcome, including poor social and emotional adjustment. Therefore there is an urgent need to address this fulminating issue, by providing educational and clinical help to both bullied and the perpetrator. I have known teenagers who committed suicide due to bullying. It is important for school communities, to have a coordinated response, for addressing bullying among youth and for families to be involved, in addition to coordinated community approach.

Schools must measure the prevalence of bullying and share the survey with school community. It may galvanise the support and understanding of people to the magnitude of the problem, and may want to assist in addressing it.

Case Study

A 13 years old teenager was referred to see me, due to her increasing isolation and school refusal. She came to live with her father soon after her mother's death. Her dad was a single and well-employed man, who was fighting for her custody, since his separation from her mother, some 8 years ago. Although his contact with his daughter was minimal, he was aware of the adverse environment she was living in. Following her parents' separation, my patient aged 5 years moved in with her mother and her boyfriend, both of whom were actively involved with the underworld drug trafficking. There was significant domestic violence to which she was exposed, and was often a victim. From the age of about 8 years her stepfather started to, sexually abuse her. She was kept out of school, and was not allowed to visit any of the family members. In one of incidence of domestic violence, she received serious facial injuries requiring multiple operations. The situation continued for nearly 3 years when her mother died of an overdose and with the help of the Department of Community Services her father was able to bring her home. His commitment and dedication to his daughter was exemplary. He gave up his job to take care of his daughter who required ongoing medical care for the injuries she received.

Her experience in the local school was traumatic. She suffered from, social anxiety, panic attacks and agoraphobia, which made her vulnerable to victimisation. This was her experience in 2 local public and 1 private schools. She was not included in any group. Although she was a beautiful looking teenager, she was self-conscious of the scars of her injury. She believed that her peer group talked about it. She felt discriminated as she felt that they were aware of her background. Both her father and myself wrote letters, to the schools, who were cooperative. Unfortunately at the student level nothing much changed. She was subjected to derogatory remarks discouraging her from attending school. I then successfully applied for home schooling, which she was able to continue without any fear of intimidation by her peer group. She was an intelligent, articulate, ambitious and a likeable teenager who had dreams of going to university, as a payback to her father's unconditional love.

Her vulnerability for victimisation obviously resulted from her severe childhood trauma, though she still impressed me as resilient, mature, and a highly motivated person, who had the potential for success, which I continued to reinforce to build her confidence.

Disruptive Behaviour

Disruptive behaviour of preschool years, generally settles during preadolescent years, though in some children it may not, which must be addressed to prevent disrupted schooling, deviant peer relationships, drug misuse, relationships, employment and stress management of adult life (Robins Lee). Childhood conduct disorder is an accurate predictor of adult criminality even up-to 30 years later. The good news is that early intervention can reverse or deliver promising results by combining parents, teachers and dedicated mental health professionals.

ADHD

Attention-deficit/ hyperactivity disorder (ADHD): Is not an uncommon diagnosis, which has become increasingly well known over the past 5 decades.

A neuropsychiatric condition characterized by functional impairment due to persistent inattention, impulsivity and motor restlessness sufficient to interfere with social and academic functioning.

However it will only be fair to outline the ongoing controversy in the existence of ADHD. There has been emotive and sensationalist debate between those that promote core belief in ADHD and those who do not. Large number of greater than chance comorbid conditions encountered in young people with ADHD present clinical and research dilemmas.

DSM, and ICD have only been moderately successful in establishing the diagnostic reliability. National institute of Mental Health's Research Domain Criteria (RDoC), which are to be based on underlying biological components conceptualised as disorders in brain circuitry, may offer 'promising greater reliability of diagnosis' (F Levy. 2014).

ADHD is primarily driven by developmental delay biologically, psychologically and socially. Many genes of small effect interact with, and are modulated by environmental factors (NICE 2009). Extensive literature shows that genetic and neurobiological underpinnings are responsible for the symptoms as well as clinical impairment in several life areas, which can be mitigated with pharmacological and psychosocial approaches (Faraone SV 2005).

It co-occurs at substantially high rate with oppositional defiant behaviour, which has features of defiance, hostility and negativism. The two together can lead to dangerous behaviour in adulthood, such as conduct disorder or substance abuse.

A high prevalence of Vitamin D deficiency in pregnancy and neonates has been reported worldwide, and has been linked to ADHD. While the impact on bone growth and mineralisation has been known for more than century, more recent research has focused on extra skeletal manifestations of deficient vitamin D, in children. Recent findings include association between levels of maternal vitamin D during pregnancy, psychomotor functions and language development in infants and children (Morales E, et al 2015).

Supplementation of vitamin D during pregnancy is likely to reduce the risk of developing ADHD symptoms in toddlers.

ADHD is common in population of adults with substance use disorder. A meta-analysis indicated 23.1% subjects, with substance use disorder met the criteria of co morbid ADHD. The combination results in high risk of severe emotional and interpersonal problems. Both ADHD and substance abuse have reciprocal vulnerability. Stimulant medications are successfully used in childhood ADHD, which can lead to self-medication as an adult. However there is limited evidence of any benefit of psycho-stimulant in adult ADHD. Prescribing of drugs of dependence to individuals with history of substance use disorder needs careful consideration.

"The rapid expansion in the use of, culturally constructed diagnosis like ADHD, together with giving children powerful stimulants medications to control their behaviour, is damning indictment of the position of children in neo-liberal cultures, rather than an indication of scientific progress" (Timimi 2009).

When the stimulants are not advisable atomoxetine a selective nor-epinephrine reuptake-inhibitor and 2 adrenergic agonists such as clonidine and guanfacine are considered an alternative or adjunctive treatment for patients with ADHD (Feldman HM, et-al. 2014).

Failing this, either due to risk factor or intolerability, Tipepidine has been suggested: still in its initial stage of testing for ADHD patients. It is non-narcotic antitussive agent for children in Japan. It significantly increases extracellular levels of monoamines like serotonin and dopamine in prefrontal cortex (Sasaki T, et al. 2014).

Non-pharmacological treatment must be considered, with or without the medications. Behaviour management strategies, addressing problematic behaviour, may have better outcome. Learning support of scholastic skills needs to be tailored around child's individual strength to enhance their self-confidence. Both positive and negative reinforcement are likely to work better in shaping the desired behaviour. Self-regulation of emotions, dealing with negative and angry feelings must be part of comprehensive management.

ADHD is considered a continuous neurodevelopmental condition that develops in childhood, and may persists in adulthood. However contemporary clinical consensus suggests that adult diagnosis of ADHD requires an accurate recall of childhood symptoms (Adler LA, et al. 2002). It may be challenging for an adult to provide collaborative information, based on recall, in clinical setting as ancillary: likely to be subjected to critical clinical judgement.

DSM 5 extends maximum age of onset of ADHD symptoms to 12 years: reducing symptom threshold to 5, after the age of 17years. There are some recent studies suggesting that adult onset ADHD is likely to be etiologically different from child onset ADHD.

Adults with ADHD have significantly raised risk of comorbidity like conduct disorder and dysthymia.

Autism Spectrum Disorder

Autism Spectrum Disorder (ASD): Defined as, cluster of life-long neurodevelopmental disorders, consisting of autistic disorder, Asperger's syndrome and pervasive developmental disorders. ASD can be disabling disorders, warranting multifaceted assessments, and interventions required in some form, across life span. It has deficits in social communication, social interactions in addition to restricted repetitive behaviour, interests and activities.

The underlying genetic, environmental and biochemical factors have been implicated in the aetiology, with more recent focus on oxidative stress. Glutathione is the most important and widespread anti-oxidant in human body. Its deficiency has been reported in many studies as the cause of ASD, which is also associated with a range of systemic abnormalities linked to low glutathione. It acts as a free radical scavenger, and helps to buffer reactive products of oxidative reactions. Its other functions include DNA repair, protein and prostaglandin synthesis, amino-acid transport and enzyme activation. Glutathione is essential for gastrointestinal and immune system functioning, and detoxification of, organic and inorganic xenobiotics, including heavy metals like mercury and lead (Kern JK, et al 2006).

It is now estimated that 10% of children with ASD have an identifiable, genetic disorder including Rett's Syndrome, Fragile X Syndrome, Tuberous Sclerosis and Angelman Syndrome (Yang 2007)

The diagnosis may be delayed till the adolescence, though the symptoms associated with ASD appear early in child's development. The diagnosis may be eclipsed by comorbid psychiatric conditions like depression, anxiety, disruptive disorders, ADHD and psychotic symptoms.

Absence of cognitive and language deficits may also delay the diagnosis, though parents may be concerned about some vague behavioural signs. The recent advent of computer based diagnostic interview for ASDs, might be the future of screening at an early intervention service.

The presence of childhood ASDs and autistic traits increased the likelihood of, psychotic experiences in early adolescence thus lending more support to common neurodevelopmental etiological basis for both psychosis and ASD conditions (Sullivan S, et al. 2013). Genes associated with autism are also associated with schizophrenia and bipolar disorders.

It is more prevalent in boys than girls.

Early diagnosis and intensive behavioural interventions are more effective in improving long-term outcome. Teaching social skills, incorporating visual aids, family involvement, rewarding treatment compliance and using child's reinforcing interests, earlier than later, could have protective influence, in preventing psychiatric comorbid conditions during adolescence (Lang R, et al. 2011). Medication specially, atypical antipsychotics, selective serotonin reuptake inhibitors and stimulants can be used with caution. Although it does not address the core deficit in ASD there is evidence of improvement in some of the associated behaviours (West et al 2009).

Epidemiology, anecdotal reports and educational and service provider statistics reveal a growing epidemic of ASDs. There has been increasing concern about the over-diagnosis, in case of it being inappropriate. It may impose unnecessary management plan, of social isolation, and qualifying for disability pension in Australia, removing the motivation to become independent (Basu S 2013). Therefore the assessment must be, comprehensive bio-psychosocial formulation that considers, all developmental and contextual factors, in a child's life, engaging child, family and school.

Adolescent Depression

Adolescent Depression: Adolescence is the most significant phase of life; a transitional stage, where young people forge their sense of identity, and start to develop their social role they hope to inhabit, in their adult life.

Depression a relatively rare diagnosis, in childhood, commonly arises, during adolescence with annual prevalence of up to 8% (Sawyer et al. 2001). Mood symptoms are most dynamic in late adolescence and early adulthood and surge to a peak between 15 and 17 years (Kessler RC, et al. 2001).

About 40% of people with diagnosis of major depressive disorder (MDD) suffered their first depressive episode before the age of 20 years and 50% adolescents, diagnosed with MDD before the age of 18 years may have further episodes of MDD during the adulthood.

Intermittent sub-threshold depressive symptoms affect 10-20% of all young people which may represent maturation process as a part of normal development (Wesselhoeft R, et al. 2013).

When people with genetically determined vulnerability are exposed to, certain internal and external environmental risk factors, they are very likely to experience chronically elevated levels of depression. Internal risk factors appear to include sex hormones (testosterone may have a protective effect) and certain cognitive and psychological traits (ruminations and negative cognitive style). External factors include chronic psychosocial stress, novelty seeking and delayed gratification. The protective factors for adolescent depression are: adequate parental support, intact family structure, favourable socio-economic status and, psychological traits, like adaptive coping and resilience.

It can cause significant burden to adolescent's relationship with family and peers, academic performance and personal development. The most tragic consequence of depression can be suicidal behaviour. Suicide is leading cause of death, among youth worldwide. Apart from mental illness, difficulties in parent child relationship, perceived low level of parental care, history of childhood abuse, exposure to recent stressful life event, academic pressure, peer victimisation and perceived body image can all cause depression and, suicidal behaviour. Early recognition of risk factors and management of adolescent's sub-threshold depressive symptoms must be promptly addressed to minimise suicidal ideations.

Interestingly both higher and lower socioeconomic status is considered risk factor for psychological stress. High-income families specially, of Asian background invest and expect high returns from the children which may be the cause of the stress and depression

Paediatric Bipolar Disorder

Paediatric bipolar disorder? A diagnosis yet to find its place in the classification of, psychiatric illnesses: for right reasons. Although bipolar illness begins, at an early age, and possibly amenable to prevention, the diagnosis can be confounding, given the dimensional nature of psychiatric diagnosis. At what stage one can pathologise a child's natural disinhibitions, temper tantrums, excitement, pressure of speech and fantasy of grandiosity?

With the research available at this stage there is no justification to formally recognise it. The concept is prematurely translated into clinical practice.

There is no consensus on its symptoms, and the accurate diagnosis may not be possible. The use of psychotropic medication with its iatrogenic dangers is not without serious risk on the developing brain, and mostly it will have dangerous potential for abuse (Malhi GS, et al. 2020).

Tourette Syndrome

Case Study

An 11 years old girl was first referred to me. She lived with her mother, stepfather and an older half sister. She was struggling at school and was teased for her jerky abnormal movements. Her symptoms of complex motor and vocal tics started about 3 years ago. Additionally she suffered from panic attacks and anxiety, which affected her schoolwork. She was overweight and had certain obsessional features like arranging things in order and difficulty in changing her thoughts. Her mother suffered from long standing depression, and panic attacks.

Her diagnosis was complex though a part of it was Tourette syndrome. There was no success with cognitive or behavioural therapy, so after consulting a child psychiatrist colleague I tried her on small dosages of antidepressants and antipsychotic medication. There was also possibility of attention deficit disorder, which could not be confirmed due to her fluctuating symptoms and response to treatment. Her home life was unsettling from the outset; a breeding ground, for psychological unrest. Her symptoms of jerky movement, motor and verbal tics improved, over the next 10 years. She irregularly contacted me with recurring symptoms of maladjustment.

Tourette Syndrome was, first described by Gilles de la Tourette in 1885. It is neurodevelopmental disorder characterised by abnormal motor movements, multiple motor tics, at least one vocal and, coprolalia, generally appearing, before the age of 18 years, and at least one year of duration. Prevalence rate 0.4% to 3.8% for children aged 5-18 years and rarely in adults (EapenV, et al. 2016).

Its association with comorbid psychiatric illnesses is around 90%. The most commonly reported are OCD, ADHD and autism spectrum disorder. Prognosis gets worse with complexity of comorbidity specially, with ADHD. Assertive management of comorbidity is indicated where these are causing distress and impairment

The symptoms generally get better with age though its persistence in adulthood is not uncommon. The treatment can be difficult. Recent trials of pharmaceutical grade cannabis, has shown some promise of success. Risperidone has also been tried with limited success. However the current available treatment is only symptomatic and not disease modifying.

Intellectual Disability

Intellectual Disability (ID): The prevalence of Intellectual disability, in Australia is estimated at 1.7%, and at higher level in low-income countries.

Although a minority group in Australia, it requires high-level care. Individuals with ID, experience substantial difficulty in everyday living, are at higher level of physical ill health, and 5-12 folds increased risk of mortality (Bourke et al 2017).

Majority have psychiatric disability; up to 3 times more than experienced by general population with over-representation of mental illnesses and earlier onset. They are at the risk of under-diagnosed and underserviced for their mental health issues due to diagnostic overshadowing.

Specific genetic conditions associated with ID and developmental brain abnormalities as well as pharmacological treatments can increase the risk of psychopathology. ID remains a neglected area with poor understanding of psychiatric illness comorbidity, both by the family and the health professionals. There is need for comprehensive service framework to improve the health care of people with intellectual disability.

Youth Social Withdrawal Behaviour

Youth social withdrawal behaviour: there is increasing evidence of young people who seclude themselves in their room, do not attend school or work and have minimal social contact. It is not only a social issue but is becoming a psychiatric issue as well. They may not fit into any psychiatric label therefore suggestions are made for severe social withdrawal to be considered as a new category of diagnostic classification. However sociologists view it as another social issue of youths. For some young people it may be the preferred life style for self-searching as long as there is social and financial support (LI TMH, et al. 2015).

Over-dependent, socially withdrawn youths grow up in overprotective families, where they may fail to develop healthy psychosocial development like autonomy and interpersonal trust. The home then becomes comfort zone reinforcing secure attachment.

The next group is likely to be maladaptive interdependent youths, also facing family issues of dysfunctional dynamics and parenting, which forms the basis of learning their interpersonal skills. This leads to their social maladjustment in the peer group, resulting in rejection and bullying.

The next group for social withdrawal comes from highly ambitious families: burdened with high expectations of the achievement-oriented parents. The pressure for performance impacts on psychosocial personal development necessary for functional adult life.

Prolonged social withdrawal may undermine the communication and interpersonal skills. Nevertheless some may continue communication via digital means.

Treatment of these youths may be challenging, as they are difficult to engage. Attempts have been made to use pet animals or internet/social media, facilitating communication and for their gradual entry into the real world.

The Productivity Commission 2020 has strongly emphasized prevention and early intervention. The proposed inclusion of social and emotional wellbeing in the existing physical examination of infants will be a welcome step forward. Appointment of a full time teacher for mental health and wellbeing in every school at the cost of 1 billion a year must be applauded as the foresight of Australian government in right direction.

References

Adler LA, Chua HC. (2002) Management of ADHD in adults. The Journal of Clinical Psychiatry 63: 29-35.

Agorastos A, Pervanidou P, et al. 2018 Early life stress and trauma: Developmental neuroendocrine aspects of prolonged stress system dys-regulation. Hormones 17: 507-520.

Aas M, Navari S, et al. 2012 Is there a link between childhood trauma, cognition and amygdala and hippocampal volume in first episode psychosis? Schizophrenia Research 137: 73-79.

Althoff RR, Verhulst FC, et al.2010 Adult outcomes of childhood dys-regulation: A14 years follow up study. Journal of the American Academy of child and adolescent psychiatry 49: 1105-1116.

Analitis F, Vederman MK, et al. Being Bullied: Associated factors in children and adolescents 8-18 years old in 11 European countries. Paediatrics 2009; 123: 569-577.

Basu S, Parry P. The autism spectrum disorder 'epidemic': Need for bio-psychosocial formulation ANZJP 47(12) 1116-1118.

Bateman A and Fonagy P. Randomised controlled trial of outpatient mentalisation based treatment versus structured clinical management of borderline personality disorder. Am J Psychiatry 2009; 17: 1355-1364.

Bostwick JM, Pabbati C, et al (2016) Suicide attempt as a risk factor for completed suicide: Even more lethal than we knew. American Journal of Psychiatry 173: 1094-1100.

Bourke J, Nembhard WN, et al. (2017) Twenty-five years survival of children with intellectual disability in Western Australia. The Journal of Paediatrics 188: 232-239.

Cicchetti D. 2016. Socio-emotional, personality and biological development: Illustrations from multilevel developmental psychopathology perspective on child maltreatment. Annual Review of Psychology 67:187-211.

EapenV, Sneddon C, et al. Tourette syndrome comorbidities and quality of life. ANZJP 2016.Vol 50 (1), 82-93.

Faraone SV 2005. The scientific foundation for understanding attention deficit/ hyperactivity disorder as a valid psychiatric disorder. European Child and Adolescent Psychiatry14: 1-10.

Feldman HM and Reiff MI. 2014. Attention deficit hyperactivity disorder in children and adolescents. New England Journal of Medicine370: 838-846.

Glaser, Portegijs et al (2006) Childhood trauma and emotional reactivity to daily life stressors in adult. Journal of psychosomatic Research61: 229-236.

Green M, Tzoumakis S, et al. Latent profiles of early developmental vulnerabilities in New South Wales child population at age 5 years. 2018 ANZJP, Vol 52 (6) 530-541.

Guy S, Furber G et al. 2016 How many children in Australia are at risk of mental illness? ANZJP50: 1146-1160.

Johnstone E, Lawrence D, et al. Service use by Australian children for emotional and behavioural problems: Finding from the second Australian Child and Adolescent Survey of Mental Health and Wellbeing ANZJP 2016 Vol 50(9) 887-898.

Kern JK, and Jones AM. (2006) Evidence of toxicity, oxidative stress and neuronal insult in autism. Journal of Toxicology and Environmental Health. Part B: Critical Reviews. 9: 485-499.

Kessler RC, Avenevoli S, et al. 2001 Mood disorders in children and adolescents: An epidemiological perspective. Biological Psychiatry 49: 1002-1014.

Lang R, Mahoney R, et al. Evidence to practice: treatment of anxiety in Individuals with autism spectrum disorder. Neuropsychiatr Dis Treat 2011; 7: 27-30.

Lawrence D, Johnson S, et al (2015) The mental health of children and adolescents. Report on the 2nd Australian Child and Adolescent Survey of Mental Health and Well-being. www.health. gov. au/internet/main/ publishing. nsf./ child2. Pdf.

Levy F (2014) DSM-5, ICD-11, RDoC and ADHD diagnosis ANZJP 48: 1163-1169.

LI TMH, Wong PWC. Youth social withdrawal behaviour: A systematic review of qualitative and quantitative studies. ANZJP 2015; Vol 49(7) 595-609.

Liotti G. Trauma, disassociation and disorganised attachment: three strands of a single braid. Psychotherapy: Theory, Research, Practice, Training 2004; 41:472-486.

Lui X. 2004 Sleep and adolescent suicidal behaviour. Sleep 27: 1351-1358. Malhi GS, Bell e, et al. Paediatric Bipolar Disorder: pre-pubertal or premature ANZJP2020 Vol 54 (5) 547-550.

Mathews R, Hall WD, et al. (2011) What are the major drivers of prevalent disability burden in young Australians. MJA 194:232-235.

Morales E, Julvez J, et al 2015. Vitamin D in pregnancy and attention deficit hyperactivity disorder-like symptoms in childhood. Epidemiology 26: 458-465.

National Institute for Health and Clinical Excellence (NICE) 2009 Attention Deficit Hyperactivity Disorder: The NICE guidelines on diagnosis and management of ADHD in Children, Young People and Adults. Leicester: The British Psychological Society and The Royal College of Psychiatrists

Nazarov A, Frewan P, et al. 2014. Theory of mind performance in women with post-traumatic stress disorder related to childhood abuse. Acta Psychiatrica Scandinavica 129:193-20.

Robins, Lee Deviant Children Grown Up: A sociological and psychiatric study of sociopathic personality 1974. Amazon.com.

Sasaki T, HashimotoK, et al. 2014. Tipepidine in children with attention deficit hyperactivity disorder: a 4 weeks, open label, preliminary study. Neuropsychiatric Disease and Treatment 10: 147-151.

Sawyer MG, Arney FM et al. The mental health of young people in Australia: key findings from the child and adolescent component of national survey of health and wellbeing. ANZJP 2001; 35: 806-814.

Scott J and Moore S, et al. 2014. Bullying in children and adolescents: a modifiable risk factor for mental illness ANZJP 48: 209-212.

Stanford S, Jones M, and et al. Understanding women who self harm: Predictors and long-term outcomes in a longitudinal community sample. (2017) ANZJP Vol 51(2) 151-160.

Sullivan S, Rai D, et al. The association between autistic spectrum disorder and psychotic experiences in the Avon longitudinal study of parents and children (ALSPAC) birth cohort. J Am Acad Child adolesce Psychiatr 2013; 52; 806-814.

Timimi S and Leo J (eds) 2009 Rethinking ADHD: From Brain to Culture. Basingstoke: Palgrave MacMillan

van Dam DS, van der Van E et al. Childhood bullying and the association with psychosis in non-clinical and clinical samples: A review and meta-analysis. Psychol Med 2012; 42: 2463-2474.

Wesselhoeft R, Sorensen, et al. 2013. Sub-threshold depression in children and adolescents: A systematic review. Journal of Affective Disorder 151: 7-22.

West L, Waldrop J, et al. (2009) Pharmacologic treatment for the core deficit and associated symptoms of autism in children. Journal of Paediatric Health Care 23: 75-89.

Yang MS and Gill M (2007) A review of gene linkage, association and expression studies in autism and an assessment of convergent evidence. International Journal of Developmental Neuroscience 25: 69-85.

PERSONALITY DISORDER

A SERIOUS, SEVERE AND complex mental disorder associated with, high cost. Globally it is estimated to affect 6% of population and yet, its not recognised for its personal and widespread damage. Personality disorders have been excluded, when reporting on mental health morbidity (Tyrer P, et al. 2010).

In Australia, within its Medicare scheme there is no specified avenue for treating personality disorder. Evidence based psychological treatment is recommended for long-term recovery specially, before the age of 18 years. Unfortunately, it is low in the list of available psychiatric workforce.

DSM-5 describes it as an enduring pattern of inner experiences and behaviour that deviates markedly from the expectations of the individual culture, causing clinically significant distress in most areas of significant functioning. It causes more grief and challenge to both, patient and the therapist as well as people around. Dimensional approach to personality attributes must distinguish between functional and pathological traits. There is evidence of genetic vulnerability, which interacts with noxious environmental experiences disrupting fundamental processes associated with personality development.

ICD-11 represents a radical change from ICD-10 classification. Individual categories of personality disorders have been removed and replaced by a core diagnosis of personality disorders, which may be specified as mild, moderate or severe.

Borderline Personality Disorder (BPD): I find difficult to separate BPD from Complex PTSD. Although complex PTSD is not included in DSM-5, ICD-11 included it as enduring personality change after catastrophic experiences (Resick PA 2012). Within mental health setting, approximately 10% of all psychiatric outpatients and between 15-25% of psychiatric inpatients meet the criteria of BPD (Leichsenring, et al. 2011).

With 5.9% lifetime prevalence, it is a common debilitating and highly stigmatised illness characterised by persistent and pervasive cognitive, affective and behavioural dys-regulation resulting in emotional instability, difficulty forming relationships and self-destructive behaviour. There are 4 core elements for BPD (Mears R, et al 2011a).

'Painful incoherence' (highly intense emotional pain reflecting a fragmented sense of self; the most significant factor)

'Inconsistency'

'Role absorption' (loss of identity)

'Lack of commitment' (least significant)

In terms of aetiology, the bio-psychosocial model of BPD postulates that early signs of emotional hypersensitivity coupled with poor emotional control interact with exposure to an invalidating care giving environment (disrupted attachments and childhood neglect and abuse), shaping the individual's marked emotional ability, leading to maladaptive coping strategies (Parker G, et al. 2018).

Impulsive personality disorder traits are independently higher in relatives of those with BPD predicting the role of gene-environment interactions including, temperamental vulnerability.

Strong countertransference reactions including anger, frustration and indifference, are commonly reported by clinicians working with BPD specially, in context of drug and alcohol abuse (Bourke ME, et al. 2013).

My training barely mentioned BPD though the kind of patients of this category did exist and were recognised by different labels midway between neurosis and psychosis. BPD was first included in 1980 edition of DSM-3. Following this Stevenson and Meares in 1992 published, the findings on successful psychotherapy for Borderline Personality Disorder (BPD), which opened the doors for its exploration and wider recognition as an independent diagnosis. There has been some controversy about its inclusion with other personality disorders due to its significant history of abuse and trauma as a child in the background.

One of the significant reasons for the misdiagnosis has been; presence of auditory verbal hallucinations, which is part of at-least ¼ if not half of BPD patients, impacting on its treatment and outcome. As there is remarkable history of childhood sexual abuse and neglect in BPD, the hallucinations are considered dissociative and are more likely to be related to the abuse. In addition to auditory hallucinations, commanding self-harm and making derogatory remarks, the patients can also experience olfactory, tactile and visual hallucinations. It is important to separate the symptoms of BPD from Schizophrenia due to different treatment modalities for the 2 illnesses. Hallucinations in BPD are generally triggered by stress. Thought disorder and negative symptoms are either minimal or absent. Presence of positive psychotic symptoms may be poor prognostic indicators.

Affective responses generally appear appropriate, and BPD patients retain sociability.

Apart from their poor self-care, people with BPD are prone to comorbidity for psychiatric, drug misuse and physical illnesses, complicating their management. Inability to control their emotions specially internalised anger, low stress threshold and impulsivity makes them more vulnerable to self-injury, suicidal thoughts and high-risk sexual behaviour. They mostly cope with stress by overwhelming sense of despair and helplessness, resulting in intense and exaggerated feelings of depression, and its neural correlates of hyperactive amygdala (Schulz L, et al. 2016).

Repeated episodes of emotional crises are characteristic of BPD, which may also trigger reactive depression though profound experience of sadness may not always be part of depressive syndrome. Negative self-concept and self-loathing as an intrinsic factor, leads to self-damaging behaviour.

Although mostly victimised and exploited, they can act violently with prospect of abandonment, which was first described by Masterson as borderline construct. It may have its origin in early insecure attachment (Bowlby J. 1988).

Caregiver's responsiveness and proximity, shapes infant security and bonding, with long-term implications for future relationships on multiple domains.

BPD patients do not like limit settings and boundaries around the availability of their therapist. They show capacity to form intense though meaningful relationship with their therapist.

The relationship between BPD and bipolar affective disorder and the confusion leading to its misdiagnosis have been a continuous debate, due to some common symptoms. Cyclothymic temperament, rapid cycling mood and self-injury, may be, the shared character between the two. Family history in bipolar disorder is more prominent than in BPD. Deficits in cognitive functions are more severe in bipolar disorder and less generalized in BPD (Kurtz MM, et al 2009). There are likely to be more suicide attempts by borderline patients against more completed suicide among bipolar patients.

During an episode of acute illness, patients with bipolar disorder may exhibit affective instability, impulsivity, explosive rage, manipulative interpersonal behaviours, self-injury, which may also lead, to the diagnosis of BPD (Tiller JW 2010).

An interesting hypothesis has been forwarded of endogenous opioid dysfunction, which can explain some of the emotional symptoms, of BPD (Bandelow B, et al. 2010).

Neuro-biologically the loss of grey and white matter is more pronounced in bipolar than BPD. Overall there seems to be evidence for fronto-limbic dysregulation in both bipolar and BPD, though the latter has more disruption of functional network connectivity specially the amygdala. Although they share many clinical and biological signs including pathophysiology and psychopathology, the evidence suggests that they remain essentially distinct entities and may co-occur (Darryl Basset.2012).

BPD is overrepresented in clinical and forensic samples of patients who have histories of violent behaviour and crimes (Gonzalez R, et al 2016).

Patients with comorbid borderline and antisocial personality disorder have more criminal conduct, more substance abuse, police contact and self-reported violence and reoffend more often after release from prison. BPD has greater impact on female violence largely due to unstable relationships (Freestone M, et al. 2013).

Like most psychiatric patients, BPD patients are prone to react negatively, to any criticism, which they internalise, undermining their self worth and impacting on their treatment outcome. Therefore one of the treatment goals must aim to return them to a more fulfilling life like social activities, education and employment. Recovery should not only be limited to symptom removal but discovering a meaningful and satisfying life, harnessing resilience.

Long term Psychoanalytically orientated psychotherapy used to be the recommended treatment, till Dialectical Behaviour Therapy (DBT) became the gold standard therapy for BPD. It is organised around delivery of skills to manage emotional dys-regulation, self-destructive behaviour, and interpersonal problems. Unfortunately it is not easily accessible due to financial cost and dearth of trained therapists.

I have also found conversational model developed by Russel Mears (Australia) and Robert Hobson (UK) of interpersonal therapy, as well as cognitive behaviour therapy useful, in most psychiatric patients.

Mentalization based therapy in context of an attachment relationship, is also recommended for BPD. It helps the person maintain mentalizing within interpersonal context before it is lost, so that emotional dys regulation, self destructive behaviour and interpersonal problems are controlled and do not cascade towards the non mentalizing process resulting in the prototypical behaviours of BPD.

Transference Focused Psychotherapy is, structured, twice weekly, psychodynamic evidence based treatment, for severe personality disorders particularly BPD. As the subjective and interpersonal experiences are often exaggerated and distorted, the aim is to use the activation of this in the treatment relationship, to frame the affect cognitively that arise in relationships, in order to facilitate integration of the related conflicting internal object relations in to more cohesive and functional personality structure (Draiger N 2013)

The dissociation /childhood trauma may be relevant in considering psychodynamic psychotherapies in addressing defence mechanisms.

Pharmacotherapy has a role in the treatment but for short term and largely symptomatic. Multidisciplinary management is preferred to minimise the transference and countertransference between the patient and the therapist.

Spontaneous improvement is common by the fourth decade; till than harm minimisation must remain the priority (Bassett D. 2017.).

Burden of BPD outweighs other psychiatric disorders. The National Health and Medical Research Council of Australia recently estimated that 23% of outpatient and 43% of inpatient mental health service users have a diagnosis of BPD.

Case Study

A 28 years old, single woman was referred by her general practitioner, as she was about to lose, the custody, of her new born child. This was her third child. The older 2 children were, adopted by her mother and her aunt. She had long history of unsettled life dating back to her early adolescence. She was expelled from school around the age of 13 years for selling illicit drugs to her fellow students. After about 6 months at home, without any goal or purpose and on her parents' insistence, she was accepted back at school. Her next 12 months were traumatic. She felt miserable, both at school and at home, with repeated threats of suicide. Her friend confided in her of slashing her wrist, for comfort, which she copied. Once her family found out she was taken to hospital casualty.

She subsequently left school at the age of 15 years and had her first child at 16 years of age. Following an argument with her family she left home and found a group of homeless teenagers sharing an abandoned house. She started using illicit drug though luckily found a drug counselor who helped her return home. She could not bond with her daughter who was under care of her mother. Feeling alone and rejected she had another child in the hope of starting a family. Unfortunately the unstable relationship with her boyfriend ended and she lost interest in the baby who was adopted by her aunt. This was followed by few more attempts of suicide by overdoses and cutting her legs and arm. In between she did attempt a few casual jobs but not for long.

I was unable to support her case for taking care of her child, which made her angry. I suggested, that I need to see her regularly for a few months before supporting her application which was not possible as she was continuously involved in one or other critical event like finding a new boyfriend, and becoming pregnant once again. She finally agreed to keep her appointment. Unfortunately, the night before, she was arrested by the police for carrying certain amount of cannabis, in her car and driving under influence of alcohol.

Women with BPD, experience higher level of parenting stress, and far less satisfaction with parenting. They are less sensitive and more intrusive. Infants with BPD mothers have increased risk of insecure attachment style, ADHD and conduct disorder. They suffer from poor emotional regulation and negative expectations of their parents, as well as fear of abandonment (Newman L K, et al. 2007).

The interesting, curiosity will be; as what happens to BPD diagnosed patients as they get older. Although reliable data are still scant, it seems that the core features of impulsivity like suicidality and deliberate self harm resolve with ageing. However the temperamental symptoms like chronic dysphoria, emptiness, dependency-issues, fear of, abandonment, countertransference and anger are more persistent. Frequent use of somatisation often expressed in demands of medical attention, defiance of rules, inconsiderate behaviour and disturbed interpersonal relationships, can cause significant psychosocial stress within the person and the people around. Self-perpetuating and attention seeking behaviour can compromise any effective care by the family as well as by the professional carers (MorganTA, 47).

References

Bandelow B, SchmahlC et al. 2010 A dys regulation of the endogenous opioid system? Psychological Review 117:623-636.

Bassett D. Personality disorders: a Retrospective ANZJP 2017. Vol 51(7) 658-659.

Bourke ME, Grenyer BFS Therapist accounts of psychotherapy process associated with treating patients with borderline personality disorder J Pers Disord 2013; 27:735-745.

Bowlby J. A secure-base. Parent-child attachment and healthy human development New York: Basic Books, 1988.

Darryl Basset. Borderline personality disorder and bipolar affective disorder. Spectra or spectre? A review. 2012 ANZJP, 46 (4) 327-339.

Draiger N and Van Zon P. Transference focussed psychotherapy with former child soldiers: meeting the murderous self. J Trauma Dissoc 2013;14: 170-183.

Freestone M, Richard R, et al. Adult antisocial syndrome comorbid with borderline personality disorder is associated with severe conduct disorder, substance dependence and violent anti sociality. Personal Mental Health 2013; 7: 11-21.

Gonzalez R, Igoumenou, et al Borderline personality disorder and violence in the UK: categorical and dimensional trait assessment. BMC Psychiatry 2016; 16: 180.

Kurtz MM, Gerraty RT 2009 A meta-analytic investigation of neurocognitive deficit in bipolar illness: Profile and effects of clinical state. Neuropsychology 23: 551-562.

Leichsenring F Leibing E, et al. (2011) Borderline personality disorders The Lancet 377: 74-84.

Mears R, Gerul F, et al 2011a. Is self-disturbance the core of borderline personality disorder? An outcome study of borderline personality factors ANZJP 45: 214-221.

Morgan TA, Chelminski I, et al. Differences between older and younger adults with borderline personality disorder on clinical presentation and impairment. Journal of Psychiatric Research 47: 1507-1513.

Newman L K, Stevenson C et al. Borderline personality disorder, mother infant interaction and parenting perception: Preliminary findings. ANZJP 2007; 41: 598-605.

Parker G, McCaw S, Bayes Adam. Borderline personality disorder: does its clinical features show specificity to differing developmental risk factors? Australasian Psychiatry March 2018.

Resick PA, Bovin MJ, et al. A critical evaluation of complex PTSD literature: Implications for DSM-5. J of Traumatic Stress 2012; 25:241-251.

Schulz, L Schamahi C. Neural correlates of disturbed emotion processing in borderline personality disorder: a multi modal meta-analysis. Biolo Psychiatry 2016; 79. 97-106.

Tiller JW 2010. Bipolar disorder: Diagnostic issues MJA 193:S5-9.

Tyrer P, Mulder R, et al. 2010 Personality Disorder: A new global perspective. World Psychiatry. 9:56-60.

PSYCHIATRY OF OLD AGE

ALTHOUGH IT HAS been brewing up in the other parts of the world as a sub speciality, did not land in Australia during my training period. Its RANZCP section, was established in 1987, gaining faculty status in 1999. This was followed by, mandatory training part of the Fellowship program, as well as, a certificate of advanced training. With improved health and life expectancy, both physical and mental health issues are becoming more obvious. There are age related biological, psychological, social and developmental factors. There are issues related to cognitive decline, grief and loss, resilience, physical illnesses, vulnerability, role changes as well as residential and end of life care.

Late life suicide is a growing public health concern which peaks between 60-64 years and again between 90-94 years. It is important to understand the psychological sufferings and the family dynamics. Engaging and joining the family in improving the communication and minimising the dissonance will be essential for better outcome.

With the growing number of older people, there is also increase in their forensic contribution, leading to significant rise in prison population and need for specialised care.

Dementia

Dementia: the single greatest cause of disability in Australia, over the age of 65years, the third leading cause of disability burden overall, and the second leading cause of death in Australia. Life expectancy is increasing, and older people are living much longer, where the prevalence of dementia is likely to be more than 20%. Projection in Australia by 2030 is of, higher incidence of mental disorder in those over the age of 65 years.

Alzheimer's Disease

Most of us will encounter at least one patient with **Alzheimer disease** during our career. It is increasingly prevalent with advancing age, up to 30% after the age of 65 years. It can be challenging with its symptoms of anxiety, depression and behavioural changes, and seemingly psychotic symptoms, which may dominate the underlying, slow progression of a dementing process. Pseudo-dementia (Kiloh LG. 1957:) and pseudo-melancholia (Parker G Pseudo-melancholia.2020), can lead to incorrect false diagnosis, inappropriate treatment and illness prolongation.

The typical amnestic symptoms and episodic memory impairment begin insidiously and progress gradually. It is more common in women specially, after the age of 80 years. The risk factors are primarily related to atherosclerotic cardiovascular diseases. Hypertension, diabetes, smoking, obesity, low education, physical and mental inactivity, and depression are some of these factors.

There are, range of hypothesized pathophysiological changes, beginning well before, the clinical symptoms become evident. The complexity and the multisystem involvement continue to explore the amyloid cascade hypothesis, and autosomal dominant familial AD, to gain better understanding of the illness.

There is consensus that early diagnosis and management of dementia improves quality of life and delays residential care placement.

Pharmacological treatment for cognitive symptoms is based upon use of acetyl-cholinesterase inhibitors and the NMDA antagonist, memantine. Although these are not disease modifying therapies: can be considered when potential benefit may outweigh the risk. Behavioural and psychological approaches are preferred with better results. Judicious and symptomatic drug treatment can be considered in some cases. There is small but statistically significant benefit, of using off–label second generation, antipsychotic medication, for the management of behavioural symptoms associated with dementia. It should be monitored for safety and efficacy.

Bone marrow derived mesenchymal stem cells animal preparations have shown some promise in the reduction of beta amyloid deposits, which could serve as a basis of stem cell therapy in AD patients (Soleimani M 2009).

Lewy Body

Dementia with Lewy bodies is a common degenerative dementia second to the incidence of Alzheimer's disease. There is more evidence of visuo-spatial, attention, and fronto-executive dysfunction, and less memory dysfunction. Visual hallucinations can be prominent early in the disease and the cognitive functions can fluctuate.

Frontotemporal-dementia

It generally has its onset well before the age of 65years. Although memory may not alter significantly, there are likely to be personality and behavioural changes. Due to atrophy of frontal and temporal lobes, the executive functions like emotional reactivity, abstract thinking, planning and organisations are first to be impaired. Language difficulties extend to speech, reading and writing. There may be increased anxiety and preoccupation with health problems.

20-30% patients have a family history.

The recommended dementia screening along with CT, MRI, SPECT and PET can be used as diagnostic investigations.

Common to the diagnosis of dementia in general, there is no disease modifying treatment. General dementia care along with symptomatic treatment and judicious use of psychotropic medications is best advised.

Huntington's Disease

Profoundly incapacitating, progressive neurodegenerative disorder usually, beginning in midlife, with characteristic triad of, motor, cognitive and neuropsychiatric symptoms. The main focus of the disease is on the family history, being transmitted as an autosomal-dominant trait with high penetrance. Genetic testing is also available in prenatal planning via chorionic villus sampling and amniocentesis and, in conjunction with in vitro fertilization (de Die-Smulders, et al. 2013).

As for neuropathology there are neural losses leading to generalized cerebral atrophy. Gradual atrophy of striatum due to neural loss is the hallmark.

The prodromal symptoms may not be noticeable, or misdiagnosed, delaying the diagnosis. Behavioural, psychiatric and emotional symptoms like affective disturbances can precede the classical motor symptoms by many years. Subtle abnormal, clumsy and awkward movements can also predate the more disabling symptoms of involuntary movements and chorea. Cognitive symptoms of HD primarily reflect a form of subcortical dementia characterized by memory deficit, psychomotor slowing and impairment in executive, perceptual and spatial skills (Paulson JS. 2011).

As the disease progresses the ability to communicate diminishes. Common speech difficulties like dysarthria with poor articulation and slurring of words, slow production of words, poor speech initiation, and difficulty organizing thoughts, sets in place. Along with this there is bradykinesia, rigidity, dystonia and increased muscle tone resulting in joint contracture. Chorei-form movements persist specially, in the extremities and orobuccal region. Double incontinence and cachexia becomes manifest.

Unfortunately there is no disease modifying current therapy for HD. The treatment has to be symptomatic, support and ultimately institutional care.

Case Study

A 35 years old mother of two young children was living with her husband working as a school-teacher. She developed vague fluctuating mild symptoms which she ignored till her clumsiness was noticed by her family. Over the next 12 months she developed jerky involuntary movements and finally decided to give up her work. I was contacted by, her sister as her family was not given any information or reason for the silence on the other side. She was steadily becoming more cognitively impaired to assert herself and was controlled by her husband. Her sister was aware of the family history of Huntington's-Disease, which the husband was not; and wanted to be involved in her investigations, diagnosis and management. She had understandable anxiety and fear of its possible transmission to other members of the family, now and for the future. Unfortunately she needed legal intervention for visitation rights and her appropriate involvement in the care of her sister. This also gave her an opportunity to educate the younger members of the family, alerting them to the prodromal symptoms of the disease.

She was placed in residential care as she became physically and mentally incapacitated and finally passed away 3 years later.

References

de Die-Smulders, de Wert GM, et al. Reproductive options for prospective parents in families with Huntington's disease: clinical psychological and-reflections. Hum Reprod update 2013; 19: 304-315.

Kiloh LG. Pseudo-dementia. Acta Psychiatr Scand. 1957:36336-351.

Parker G Pseudo-melancholia. Australasian Psychiatry.2020 June.

Paulson JS. Cognitive impairment in Huntington Disease: diagnosis and treatment. Curr Neurol Neurosci Rep 2011; 11:474.

Soleimani M and Nadri s 2009 A protocol for isolation and culture of mesenchymal stem cells from mouse bone marrow. Nature Protocols 4: 102-106.

THE PATHWAYS, THE PROGRESS AND THE REFINEMENTS

IT MAY NOT have direct and most obvious role of treating my patients but I have added this chapter because of its significant impact on my knowledge and practice of psychiatry over the past five decades.

Psychiatry more than any other branch of medicine is still on the trial and error stage defining definitions, diagnosis, treatments and its delivery to the patients.

According to the Australian Institute of Health and Welfare, in any given year, approximately 4 million people experience mental disorder and only 46% seek treatment. It is estimated that 3% of the population have severe and complex mental illness, yet only 1.1% of population receive clinical mental health care. Mental health spending at 9 billion per annum is at record level, almost 8% of total health budget (Australian Institute of Health and Welfare.2018).

Despite investments, generous funding, committed and highly qualified work force, the timely and appropriate help to mentally ill people is staggering.

There has been no dearth of Australia wide inquiries (at-least 32 in past 10 years), awareness campaigns, and Royal Commissions, over most of my working life albeit, with little progress.

It is well established that 75% serious mental illnesses, as well as drug and alcohol abuse emerge before the age of 25 years, which emphasizes early prevention.

Australian National Health Survey reported no decline in the prevalence of national psychological distress. On the contrary it found increased youth suicide rates, despite major increases in the use of mental health services between 2001-2018. Of 183 countries that submitted data, in relation to suicide in 2015, 95 countries had lower suicide rates than Australia. Homelessness, another risk factor for suicide, rated even worse in the OECD database of affordable housing, at 27th out of 30 countries. It is proposed that this failure in Australia is due to prevention gap and lack of quality of service.

Both nationally and internationally mental health services lag behind the desired criteria for success (Australian Institute of Health and Welfare).

The breakdown in mental health system is evidenced by, the presentations and management of mentally ill patient in the emergency departments of general hospitals, where more than 25% are substance related. They spend at least 8 hours and often 4 to 5 days in emergency ward against Australian government's 4-hour target for completed care in Emergency (Australasian College of Emer Med). Its not surprising that many voluntary patients needing help, leave before they can be accommodated for treatment.

OECD (Organisation of Economic Cooperation and Development) average for psychiatric bed is 71 per 100,000, population, against 41 per 100,00 in Australia. In my experience I found that it is not uncommon to send an acutely ill patient in the dark of the night, a few hundred km away to another hospital after searching for a bed, across the state. It is now a well-accepted fact, that in-patient public hospitals services are only used for safety and crisis stabilisation rather than for therapeutic benefit. With limited access to public psychiatric beds many patients have been caught in the nexus of care and punishment. It is driven by the needs of the organisation rather than patient. Although private hospitals cater for longer duration of hospitalisation, it is limited by the insurance companies, for specified days, generally under a month and restrictions on readmission within a month. The mean duration of hospitalisation in an Australian study was 15 days: insufficient for meaningful psychiatric treatment in most cases (Zhang J, et al. 2011). It is therefore vital to make the best possible utilisation of this limited facility by introducing not only drug treatment but psychological treatment as well. Hospitalisation is not only expensive for the health services but traumatic for the patients too.

Working under these conditions undoubtedly affects not only the doctor, responsible for the care of acutely ill patient in emergency, but patients, their families and other clinicians. Expectations of providing high quality care and not being able to deliver, is the recipe for burnout. High efforts, combined with, low rewards is emotionally exhausting and demoralising, adversely affecting the outcome (Seigrist J et al. 2016).

Australian College of Emergency Medicine (ACEM) following its national summit in 2018 highlighted, the need for urgent reforms in care of mentally ill people who are resource intensive. An inpatient psychiatric bed in Australia carries a cost of about $ 933 per day and the cost of ECU are substantially higher (https://acem.org.au).

ACEM recommended that a large proportion of community funding must be directed towards emergency mental health.

Emergency Psychiatry

Emergency psychiatry is becoming increasingly visible which may justify its division into a sub-speciality, of which the ED embedded-units, may become an integral part.

High stimulus ED is not the best destination, for a patient suffering from acute mental health crises. In 2013, NSW Ambulance (NSWA) attended over 60,000 calls that were identified by the call taker as being about a mental health problem. NSWA trains paramedics for mental health emergencies but not diagnosis or treatment.

Mental Health Acute Assessment team joined by NSWA Extended Care Paramedic, and Mental Health Clinic Nurse Consultant, with their specialised training, responds to mental health emergencies, making a joint decision for the most suitable care for the patient. The options include ED for standard psychiatric emergency care, direct transport to mental health facility, alternate mental health provider, or to leave patient at home with follow up visits (Faddy SC. 2017).

One of the first Psychiatric Emergency Care Center (PECC), a purpose built unit opened in 2007, as part of The Nepean Hospital in Penrith NSW (Australia), adjacent to emergency department. It has maximum patient stay of 48 hours followed by transfer to acute psychiatric unit if required. The follow up results of the unit, after eight years, reported overall reduction, in admission rates, use of chemical or physical restraints and length of stay. There was increase in the diagnosis of borderline personality disorder. These encouraging outcome, resulted from education provided, to the staff around diagnostic practices, adherence to admission criteria and training of ED medical officer on mental health act (Seymour J, et al.2020).

Another version of care model Psychiatric Assessment and Planning Units (PAPUs) were built in Melbourne Australia within close proximity of ED, comprising 6-8 beds to provide recovery orientated, person centered care. It includes differentiated specialist model of care, improved system efficiency, reduced ED mental health wait times and overall improved quality of care for patients presenting in crisis. Timely and short-term in-patient care, up to 72 hours reduces demand on the ED staff (Mitchell DA, 2020).

Unfortunately, neither of these units is equipped to manage, the high-risk patients and those with extreme behavioural disturbances.

Extension of program like PECC and PAPUs can be used as simulation based medical education to improve the knowledge, skills and attitude of ED doctors in assessment of psychiatric presentations. The realistic involvement of real people and their real stories create an engaging and powerful education tool.

There was widespread criticism through media, in the recent years, of the declining public mental health services and generally against psychiatry. Increasing number of psychiatrists were leaving public sector to join private practice, of whom, more were concentrated in select metropolitan areas. It is true that unless needing acute hospitalization, patients receive better and more personal service in the private sector. As an essential domain of Australian psychiatry, private practice cannot be ignored. Time has come when private practice should be, part of training program for psychiatrists. The induction can include business planning, and practice management as foundation, building into broader leadership and management skills, as well as other modes of practice like occupational psychiatry, consulting, civil, medico-legal work and tele-psychiatry. Establishment of innovative joint network of private and public psychiatry, centered around each state College branch, may be useful, to facilitate such liaison and collaboration. Trainee psychiatrists should be encouraged to attend private practice as observers, if training position is not available (Looi JC, 2020).

Outpatient psychiatric clinics both in community and hospitals are no longer functioning for routine/regular care, which is a vital prevention strategy.

Although private psychiatric sector may be treating 50-60% people needing mental health care, we do need a public system to provide uniform care to mentally ill, irrespective of their financial status.

In talking with a senior colleague from a public hospital, I realised as how much of the special skills of a psychiatrist or a trainee, are consumed by clerical and administrative work in addition to after-hours work: a major source of dissatisfaction.

Mental health presentations to public hospital emergency department (ED) have substantially increased in the past 10 years by 50% whilst the population rose by 20%. Just half of the presentations require admission, competing for available beds.

There are, range of non-hospital mental health programs attracting funding at the expense of essential basic mental health care, which were established by the government in the hope of compensating for hospital based demands. Unfortunately these community-based programs did not provide any relief to the ED presentations. Fact remains that the crucial role of hospitals in caring for, the acutely ill, cannot be underestimated.

Constant reorganisation of public mental health services in absence of evidence, clear benefit and without evaluation, is termed as re-disorganisation which further confounds functionality of public mental health services ((Looi J, 2019). Additionally it continues to maintain the divide between administrative and clinical services.

Under the National Mental Health Strategy, the Australian government is committed to playing leadership role in setting national objectives for reforms, and measuring the progress of all governments towards them. There have been impressive national strategies and national mental health plans with ongoing collaborative framework, set goals as well as monitoring and evaluation in place. Unfortunately Australia's mental health policy lacks real accountability and relies largely on limited mental health service system data, rather than outcome data, representing a critical gap in knowledge for mental health policy, planning and practice. Mental health policy requires ongoing rigorous monitoring. The importance of outcome measurements cannot be, overstated. Even more important is, systematically measuring the experience of mental health patients, and their carers, beyond the service system (Crosbie DW. 2009).

Leadership

Ineffective governance is the key flaw, that is limiting the implementation of national mental health policy (Looi, et al.2020).

Governance challenges leading to mental health care short falls, cannot be addressed, if psychiatrists with their broad and deep expertise, are not leading and contributing, to health stewardship.

Leadership is vital in the success of any group activity. Leaders have long term vision with their eyes on the horizon and passion with which, they can enthuse those, who they wish to engage and lead. They have good communication skills and humility with wisdom. Decision-making is a vital role for the leader. For this they employ the cognitive and interpersonal skills, emotional intelligence, altruism, tenacity, strategic acumen, integrity, technical competence and expert knowledge. There is strong evidence that doctors instead of professional managers, are most closely associated with the best performing institutions, largely due to their core knowledge and experience of the organisation they are to lead. Importance of engaging doctors in planning, improving and delivering mental health care cannot be overemphasized (Goodall AH. 2015).

'Doctors need to take on leadership role-whether these are small for a team or large for an organisation or a professional body"(Bhugra 2013).

Expert leadership can translate into quality outcome. Psychiatrist executives are uniquely placed to link clinical services with academic departments of psychiatry for facilitating translational medicine. Having grown out of the same environment, doctors are more able to understand the culture, values, incentives and motivation of their colleagues.

Research should be embedded in the health system, which generates high clinical standards, benefitting patients, workforce and health care organisations. Research leadership is associated with better organisational research performance. Research focused medical leadership has been found to generate, highest performance scores in health outcomes (Ozdemir BA, et al. 2015).

National Mental Health Plans

Better Access scheme: was introduced in 2006, as the largest single component of National Action Plan for Mental Health, by the Council of Australian Government, in advance of evidence and evaluation of robust studies. Its objective was: focused psychological strategies available under Medicare. It generated almost overnight response by the prospective providers, preparing mental health plans. Its impact went as far as, psychology being the most sought after course in all Australian universities. It also allowed the psychologists to work independently rather than in multidisciplinary set up, which is required for people with complex mental health problems.

The ensuing 5 years cost to the government was, 3 times more than the initial estimate. The Budget spent on Better Access in 2010 evaluation, was nearly $500 million. Government subsequently removed access to social workers and occupational therapists under the Program. Better Access replaced Better Outcome in Mental Health Program of 2001, emphasizing the utilisation of evidence based psychological therapies for better quality of care. Unfortunately there was no detectable benefit to the mental health of Australians from the introduction of Better Access Scheme. It failed to achieve prevalence and reduction of mental illness.

'Despite considerable public funding through the Better Access scheme, there has been no demonstrable improvement in the mental health of Australians' (Jorm AF 2018).

There is also an argument in its favour that by detecting suicide risk they may have added to the increased ED presentations.

There has been substantial increase in psychological therapies, with one in every 19 Australians receiving at least one Better Access service in 2009(Perkis J, et al. 2011). However there is some evidence that users of these services are often receiving psycho-education and nonspecific counseling rather than more evidence based cognitive behavioural therapy.

Population interventions received a boost, with the start of the National Suicide Prevention Strategy in 1999, and the national depression initiative by Australian and Victorian governments in 2000, for the prevention of depression and anxiety.

Perinatal-Mental Health

Infancy is recognised as the foundation of neurological and psychological development. Therefore there is increasing attention on improving services for pregnancy, parenthood and at least for the first postpartum year.

Funding of $ 85 million from National Action plan of Australian commonwealth government to support women with depression during the pregnancy was a welcome initiative. Anxiety, depression, major life stresses and dysfunctional worry, have adverse consequences for maternal, child health and family wellbeing, both in short and long term. Preterm birth, lower birth weight and decrement in cognitive performance are some of the undesirable effects.

Perinatal period is increasingly recognised as the time of vulnerability for mental health problems. Postpartum depression is one of the most common complications of childbirth affecting both parents. Most patients with this disorder have prominent mood symptoms including anxiety, mania, mixed states and psychotic/ delusional depression as well as cognitive symptoms with similarity to those seen in bipolar episodes with intrinsically defined onset, within 4-6 weeks postpartum. The underlying neurobiological changes of endocrine, immune system and circadian rhythm occurring after child-birth, appear to be responsible for post partum symptoms.

Most of the women will recover though for some, it may herald life long course of mental illness.

Active Australasian Perinatal branch was formed in 1990. It is not only confined to the mental health of woman during pregnancy, but includes men as well for their coping skills over the transition to fatherhood. A significant number of men suffer from postpartum depression, which is detrimental to family and personal wellbeing. There is increased risk of psychiatric morbidity in the offspring of fathers who suffer from postpartum depression (Edoka et al 2010).

There are reported cases of 12 % fathers, who will follow their partner's post-partum depression (Paulson JF 2010).

Many parents experience difficulties in transition to parenthood and adaptation to the infant

Perinatal depression is now widely used term (peri-partum), which includes depression during pregnancy and after childbirth.

Anxiety disorders affect up to 15% women during pregnancy, and up to 20% in postpartum period. It can lead to obstetric complications, poor neonatal and psychosocial outcome, disruption in bonding and increased health care cost.

Depressed mothers are unable to respond, or to interact sensitively with their infant. This poor interaction, it was argued contributed to cognitive, behavioural and attachment problems, observed in the children of mothers with post-natal depression. It has long-term consequences for both: mother and the child.

High comorbidity between anxiety and depression in the perinatal period makes it imperative that treatments target both, in an effective manner (Gregoriadis S, et al. 2018). While there have been valid concerns about the safety of medication during pregnancy, anxiety and depression can also have adverse effect on the foetus and infant development (Stein A, et al 2014). Combined therapy of antidepressants and cognitive behavioural therapy is generally recommended. There is no conclusive evidence of behavioural or cognitive impairment as the result of foetal antidepressant exposure.

Epigenetic findings have shown effects of poor parenting or stress on the infant.

A focus on the family including a mentally ill women her infant and her family-has been shown not only to alleviate human cost but to provide more effective intergenerational interruption of problems and also great economic benefit with cost savings in trauma, physical and mental health, unemployment and incarceration. UK estimates suggest that for each Aus$1 invested in those critical 1001 days, Aus$10 may be saved by the time that infant reaches adolescence (Bauer A 2014). So the perinatal funding of Australian government is well timed and justified.

Interagency collaboration, to serve the individuals with persistent severe mental illness: the care coordination role of the support facilitator, as part of national **Partners in Recovery** program, was poorly received and ceased in June 2019.

Some of the other government-funded schemes include:

Headspace, Better Outcome, National Disability Insurance (NDIS) and freely available **self-help on-line therapies**: and all need caution, in their outcome results. The desired outcome must have, not only the symptom removal, but also optimal level of functioning, prevention and social support in the community as their objective.

Headspace

Youth mental health services in Australia have yet to reach the goals of investment. Headspace showed modest results underachieving its main role (Jorm AF. 2016). It was expanded without any evidence of its effectiveness. The excessive funding has been questioned for the alleged cause of depleting resources for other projects. These were some of the earlier critical reviews.

However there is renewed evidence of its progressive benefits since its inception in 2006, as it became more accessible and acceptable to young people.

In principle it was well intended in the area of high demand and necessity, but like any project, its success relies on the work practices, morale and compassion of the service providers and the strength of the leadership. It has well over 100 centers operating around the country, and plans to add another at least 50 more to provide safe, trusted, stigma free, holistic and youth friendly primary care service in partnership with local GPs. It addresses the practical hardships of vulnerable young people like accommodation, education, employment and physical and mental health. It employs community liaison staff to nurture relationships with other agencies like reaching out directly to schools and other referral points.

There is a valid argument that the existing base of public mental health services may be further enhanced by the stand-alone Headspaces specifically integrated with State/Territory mental health services (Looi et al 2020)

The debate of the Headspace investment returns aside, Prof Pat McGorry and Orygen team of Headspace was awarded historic $33 million grant in 2020, from the US National Institute of Health: an international acknowledgement of the success of the program.

National disability Insurance Scheme (NDIS)

It was first trialed in 2013 and gradually rolled out nationally over the next 4 years. There have already been concerns of misappropriation of funds and the organization has been put on alert for monitoring its fraud control processes. An estimated 4.3 million people in Australia live with disability. Over the next 5 years NDIS will provide more than 22 billion in funding to 500,000 people with permanent and significant disabilities.

Cost to Australian economy of mental ill health is, conservatively about $200 billion according to Productivity Commission Australian Government Independent Research and Advisory Body.

Many ideas come on the surface with genuine goals, of translating any new discovery for patient benefit. Spontaneous recovery needs to be considered as a valid factor in evaluating mental health funding outcome.

Medicalization of life problems beyond the bounds of evidence-based treatment may cause more problems when self-help strategies may have worked better.

References

Australasian College of Emergency Medicine. Wait times in emergency department for people with acute mental and behavioural conditions. Report ACEM. Melbourne. Available https://acem.org.au.

Australian Institute of Health and Welfare. Mental health services in Australia https//www.aihw.gov.au/reports/mental health services in Australia/ expenditure on mental health related services 2018.

Bauer A, Parsonage M, et al. The costs of perinatal mental health problems: report summary. London School of Economics, School of Mental Health, http://w w w.centreformentalhealth.org.uk/costs of perinatal-mh-problems 2014.

Bhugra D (2013) Demoralisation, deprofessionalisation, denial and detachment in medicine. ANZJP47: 1104-1107.

Crosbie DW. Mental Health Policy-Stumbling in the dark? MJA Volume 190 Number 4. Feb 2009.

Edoka IP, Ramchandani PG et al. Health care cost of paternal depression in the postnatal period. J Affect Disord 2011; 133: 356-360.

Faddy SC, Mclaughlin KJ, et al. Mental Health Acute Assessment Team: a collaborative approach to treating mental health patients in the community Australasian psychiatry 2017 Vol 25(3) 262-265.

Goodall AH, Bastiampillai T, et al. Expert leadership: doctors versus managers for the executive leadership of Australian mental health. ANZJP 2015; 49:409-411.

Gregoriadis S, Graves L, Peer M, et al. 2018 Maternal anxiety during pregnancy and the association with adverse perinatal outcome: Systematic review and meta analysis. Journal of Clinical psychiatry 74: e309-e320.

https://acem.org.au/content sources/Advancing-Emergency-Medicine/Better-Outcome-for patients.

Jorm AF Australia's 'Better Access' scheme: Has it had an impact on population mental health? ANZJP 2018. Vol 52(11) 1057-1062).

Jorm AF. Headspace: The gap between the evidence and the arguments. ANZJP 2016, Vol. 50(3) 1956-196, (NMHC 2014).

Looi JC, Atchison M. Through the looking glass: private and public practice psychiatry in the RANZCP. Australasian Psychiatry 2020 Vol 28(3) 328-330.

Looi J, Mcguire P. Australasian Psychiatry2019, Vol 27 (6) 634-636.

Looi JCL, Allison S, et al. Commonwealth of common mental health: the need for a comprehensive overhaul of corporate governance in mental health care in Australia. Australasian Psychiatry 2020 Vol 28 (3) 300-302.

Looi JCL, Allison S, et al. Response to McGorry et al,'s defence of Headspace-like Leviathans swallowing resources. ANZJP 2020 Vol 54 (11) 1059-1060.

Mitchell DA, Crawford N, et al. The efficacy, safety and acceptability of emergency embedded Psychiatry Assessment and Planning Units: An evaluation of Psychiatric Assessment and Planning Units in close proximity to their associated, emergency departments. ANZJP June 2020 Vol. 54 (6) 609-619.

Ozdemir BA, Karthikesalingam A, et al. Research activity and the association with mortality. PLoS One 2015; 10: e0118253.

Paulson J F, Bazemore S, et al. Prenatal and postpartum depression in fathers and its association with maternal depression. JAMA 2010a; 303:1961-1969.

Perkis J, Bassilios B et al.2011a Clinical improvement after treatment provided through better outcome in Mental Health Care program: do some patients show greater improvement than others? ABNZJP 45: 289-298.

Seigrist J and Li J Association of intrinsic and extrinsic components of work stress with health: a systematic review of evidence on the effort –reward imbalance model. Int J Environ Res Public Health 2016; 13: 432.

Seymour J, Chapman T, et al. Changing characteristics of a Psychiatric Emergency Care Centre. An Eight Year, follow-up study. Australasian Psychiatry. 2020 Vol 28 (3) 307-310.

Stein A, Pearson, et al (2014) Effects of perinatal mental disorder on the foetus and child. Lancet 384: 1800-1899.

Zhang J, Harvey C, et al. 2011. Factors associated with length of stay and the risk of readmission in acute inpatient facility: a retrospective study. ANZJP 45:578-585.

INTERNATIONAL RESPONSIBILITY

AS MENTAL HEALTH professionals we have a duty, to galvanise our professional bodies to raise concerns, about the mental health impacts of injustices, both in our regional neighbourhood, and in the wider world. There is estimated number of over 60 million refugees and internally displaced persons worldwide (U N Commissioner for Refugees 2014) who, commonly report an array of adverse experiences including serious, multiple and sequential traumatisation, that can involve torture, assault and traumatic loss.

Impacting on social, personal and economic consequences, immigration detention has been one of the most contentious contemporary issues, in Australia.

Onshore detention was introduced in 1992 and off shore processing started in 2001. The latter was ceased in 2007, and was reinstated in 2012 resulting in, detention of thousands of adults and children. There were multiple enquiries, providing details of widespread physical and sexual abuse, and dangerous living environment sizing up, to the criteria of United Nations' definition of torture

Australia processes 2.2% of asylum claims amongst 44 industrialised countries. In the last decade Australia granted 151,332 humanitarian visas to refugees, fleeing war, civil unrest, and political and ethnic persecutions (DIBP, 2014).

The detention of asylum seekers has been hotly debated, especially of accompanied and unaccompanied children, living in antisocial environment.

Although Australian government has passed Migration amendment for urgent medical treatment bill in 2018, it has largely preserved off shore processing as a message to future asylum seeker boats.

Asylum seekers and refugees have been held on Nauru (current number 258) and Papua New Guinea (208) for the past 7 years. Medecines Sans Frontieres (MSD): providing mental health care to this population, have reiterated their calls to end, the Australian offshore processing policy. Medevac bill, which provided transfer of the refugees to Australia, for urgent treatment was repealed by the parliament in 2019, making MSD's work even more challenging. Most of the patients under care of MSD met the criteria of depression and at least one other mental health diagnosis. 90% reported suicidal thoughts and 50% attempted suicide. New Zealand has offered to resettle, 150 refugees from Nauru and PNG every year. MSD's request, that Australia resettles the remaining asylum seekers detained within Australia or held in Nauru and PNG is still under consideration (The PULSE 2020).

Refugee Settlement

Refugee settlement is, a complex issue, often undesired and unwelcome though a moral responsibility of the stable and resourceful countries. It is much more stressful for the dislocated individual. The stress of living in a foreign culture promotes mental disorder in vulnerable individuals (Bhugra D. 2003).

The complex journey of a refugee barely finishes in one lifetime. It starts with experiences of prevailing and cumulative torture, trauma and losses in their own country and continues with the struggle of settling in a new country. Refugees are 10 times more prone to suffer from depression, anxiety, drug and alcohol excesses and post-traumatic stress disorder (Crumlish M.et al. 2010).

High rates of psychopathologies are also reported in children and adolescents from refugee background, including unaccompanied minors and are linked to, various pre and post migration risk factors (Fazel M, et al. 2012). They show poor response to treatment, which can relate to experience of disturbed interpersonal relationships, eroding their capacity to trust others and, distancing from potential attachment figures.

An estimated 200 children, seeking asylum in Australia between 2013-2019, were detained on the island of Nauru. This is very special group of children having gone through the traumatic journey from their native land to the threat of deportation from the country of their detention. Some children are detained for as long as 5 years. They not only miss out on the normal development, and healthy environment but, are subjected to, physical and sexual abuse. They witness the grief, helplessness and violence in the adult community members. Children living under unbearable life conditions can develop life threatening depression-withdrawal stress reaction. In 2017-2018, 15 children presented to MSF (Medecin Sans Frontieres) with life threatening pervasive refusal syndrome (PRS). They exhibited low mood, irritability, increasing social withdrawal, blank expression, lack of response to antidepressants, behavioural disturbance and food and liquid refusal. Some children became bed bound, mute and self-harmed (Newman L et al 2020). This I see as some of the fallacies of psychiatric treatment that a child subjected to atrocities and deprivation most of his/her life, is expected to be happy by taking antidepressants.

There was a well-publicised case I reviewed, as a Mental Health Review Tribunal member of a patient, with Australian residency and of German descent. Due to her mental illness presentation, she was misidentified, and first placed in a detention center, and than in a prison, without any treatment. Not without embarrassment though, she was finally admitted to a psychiatric unit for treatment.

Humanitarian and philanthropic roles of affluent countries have become increasingly visible and appreciated. World Health Organisation encourages collaboration of government, non-government and other organisations, to advance and promote global health, strengthening alliances in mental health system. Around 80% people living with mental illness reside in low or middle-income countries with limited access to even the inadequate resources. High-income countries spend well over 5% of their budget on mental health against 0.5% in the low and middle-income countries (Gilbert 2015).

Movement for Global Mental Health for raising the profile of mental health was established in 2014, when World Economic Forum commissioned study, identified mental illness, as the single costliest health issue, and a major barrier to the development and productivity.

The following year United Nations Department of Economic and Social Welfare included the goals of reducing premature mental health mortality by one third by 2030, broaden the scope of prevention and treatment of mental illnesses and substance abuse, and general promotion of mental health and wellbeing (Arandjelovic et al 2016).

Australia based mental health professionals and leaders have become increasingly involved in collaborating with low and middle-income countries in the last decade for improving their health services. Pacific Islands due to its proximity have become key region for Australia's support network. NSW Institute of Psychiatry has provided support and projects in the Pacific region over the past 2 decades. RANZCP in collaboration with World Psychiatric Association is progressing to develop child and adolescent mental health services within the Pacific Region, with the background, of its well developed-mental-health governance support and community services.

Working in culturally diverse settings, one has to be mindful of unintended consequences of challenging the local concepts of mental illness and replacing them with Western ones (Datta 2015).

It is also important to consider that mental health is steeped, in the social determinants of health, which are not addressed purely by mental health interventions (Kirmayer et al 2014), but by broad based community, national and international strategies

Around 2005, feeling disillusioned with life, listening to insoluble problems of my patients, almost at the verge of vicarious trauma with little recompense, I wanted to refresh myself, to regenerate the compassion and energy to positively connect with my patients again.

So I decided to take 6 months of leave. I utilised this time in starting an Eye Camp along with my husband, an ophthalmologist, in an ancient town, on the foothills of Himalaya for the under-resourced remote and rural population. I also spent 3 months at the nearby University, based on Vedic education, Dev Sanskriti in Haridwar, teaching the students of psychology.

Psychiatric Services in Fiji

Once we equipped the Eye clinic, and found like-minded professionals visiting from Australia for annual Camps, we decided to move to Fiji much closer to our home base, and poorly serviced. I accompanied my husband with his team of a dozen members to explore my possible contribution to the **mental health services in Fiji.**

I was fortunate to meet Dr Neil Sharma a medical doctor and Minister of Health. He allowed me temporary visiting role in their only psychiatric hospital, St Giles in the capitol city of Suva, with capacity of 136 beds. The two institutions of social control, a prison and a mental asylum were built in close proximity not far from the cemetery, outside the bounds of the city. My guess is that inmates and patients were interchangeable words, of the era, and the concept of reforming the 'deviants' was just emerging: a humanitarian shift from punishment to reform of those incarcerated. Pacific Island's most enduring psychiatric institution St Giles was established, as the Public Lunatic Asylum in 1884, which remained the only psychiatric facility with minimal change in the entire Pacific region till now. With nil or inaccessible mental health service, people were not even aware of such a system. They continued with their metaphysical basis of life where spirits and ancestors played an active role in illness and health, according to the conduct of people.

The colonial administration of Fiji, in their highly exploitative labour scheme, brought indentured Indian labourers to sugar farms between 1879 and 1920.

During the colonial era, Fiji became the major regional hub, as headquarter of British Western Pacific High Commission, (1877-1953) and major regional provider of health practitioner training. The introduction of psychiatric hospitalisation in 1884, a new concept, shaped Fiji's mental health services relieving the locals of their distress in caring for mentally ill people (Odille Chang. 2011).

My visit to the hospital was an eye opener with dilapidated buildings, under-resourced hospital, overworked dedicated health professionals, and outdated patient care, inconsistent with human rights. Nevertheless I was pleased to see the hospital occupational therapy section, serving well to the needs of the patients and planning to start another one in city center. I worked in outreach clinics, briefly visited psychiatric patients at home, and in the residential placements, as well as in the prison, adjacent to St Giles hospital.

I recommended, that there should be designated psychiatric beds, in the major hospitals, more affiliation with the university and improvement in the care of severely ill patients.

The Ministry of Health was able to create 5 psychiatric beds each in Suva, Lautoka and Labasa, the 3 bigger cities of Fiji, embedded in the general hospitals.

I proposed an exchange program for psychiatric nurses, which was generously supported by St John of God Hospital in Richmond NSW where I was a VMO. Unfortunately a similar program for doctors could not be created for various reasons.

I was joined by, Prof Sachdev from UNSW, Prof Raj Kumar and Dr Jagdeep Sachdev on some of the trips. We presented our project to RANZCP for collaboration and assisting Fiji in psychiatric training positions. I was grateful to Prof Sachdev for strongly supporting the proposal. Unfortunately the College was not ready at the time to venture out in the unknown territory, to consider the proposal.

It was becoming difficult to continue with the project single-handed and with the newly elected government who had other pressing items on agenda, I decided to withdraw though not without regret. I was pleased that during my last visit, Dr Odille Change the only lasting psychiatrist at St Giles hospital and totally committed to mental health, handed me a draft on Mental Health Decree for comments. Working with NSW Mental Health Review Tribunal at the time I was keen for Fiji to start similar service for their psychiatric patients. I discussed it with the president of our Tribunal who was happy to help.

Fiji Mental Health Act 1940, which was based on treating patients within the hospital, was obviously considered outdated after 70 years. So the evolution of Mental Health Decree 2010 was a welcome arrival. It promoted mental health, prevention of mental illness, community based care, rehabilitation aspects of mental health care, and human rights issues.

Although it was years later, but was pleasing to see the active involvement of Australian and New Zealand psychiatrists under the leadership of RANZCP to include Pacific Island countries in its future planning. The first issue of Australian psychiatry for the year 2020 was devoted to mental health capacity building in all its forms, to address the needs of the Indigenous Pacific communities.

The concept of Doubling emerged from a keynote presentation of Professor Omigbodun of Nigeria, then president of International Association of Child and Adolescent and Allied Professions (IACAPAP) at RANZCP Conference in 2013.

It was launched at the biennial conference of IACAPAP in Durban in 2014 to facilitate partnership between health professionals in developed high income and developing low and middle-income countries. Although RANZCP recognised it as a worthwhile initiative, and it was in accord with the College's stated aim to strengthen international relationships, their response to embrace it, was lukewarm, on the basis of several doubts. Till 2017 the College did not have a policy in respect of philanthropy or overseas support (Doubling 2019).

References

Arandjelovic K, Eyre H A, et al. Mental health system development in Asia: Does Australia has a role? ANZJP 2016 Vol 50(9) 834-841.

Bhugra D. Migration and mental health (Acta Psychiatr Scand 2003; 109: 243-258.

Crumlish M and O'Rourke K. A systematic review of treatments, for post-traumatic stress disorder, among refugees and asylum –seekers. J Nerv Ment Dis 2010; 198: 237-251.

Department of Immigration and Border Protection. Settlement reporting facility Canberra: DIBP, Australian Government, 2014.

Doubling: a model for international clinical partnerships. Australasian Psychiatry 2019, Vol 27(1) 41-43.

Datta V The problem with education in global mental health. Academic Psychiatry October 2015.

Fazel M, Reed RV, et al. Mental health of displaced and refugee children resettled in high income countries: risk and protective factors. Lancet 2012; 379: 266-282.

Gilbert BJ, Patel V, et al. 2015. Assessing development assistance for mental health in developing countries: 2007-2013. PLoS Med 12: e 1001834.

Kirmayer L J, Pederson D (2014) Towards a new architecture for global mental health. Transcultural Journal of Psychiatry 51: 759-776.

Mental Health care in Fiji by Odille Chang. Asia Pacific Psychiatry v3, n2 (June 2011): 73-75.

Newman L, O'Connor B, et al. Pervasive refusal syndrome in child asylum seekers on Nauru. Australasian Psychiatry 2020 Vol 28 (5) 585-588.

The PULSE August 2020. Medecins Sans Frontieres.

TECHNOLOGY

'Science proposes, technology executes and man conforms'
was the slogan of 1933 Chicago world Fair

'Techno society must be held responsible for the
disappearance of tranquillity, and conjure up vision of
a civilisation, totally dependent upon, and dominated
by, things technical' (Tranquillity Denied 1976).

DESPITE THE GRIM view of technology till the last century, it has
grown exponentially.

Expansion of research possibilities in the ever-increasing world of
technology, enhancing the scale of new information, and expanding the
domain of traditional and practical medicine, has opened new frontiers
in mental health care, for accessing help and education. It needs to be in
the priority health agenda of any country. In Australia, main funding
bodies for research and technology, supported by the government,
are National Health and Medical Research council, The Medical
Research Future Fund and Medical Research Endowment Account.
We need to expand graduate education, to include translational science,
entrepreneurship, business leadership and technology development, for
which we must be supported, by the funding bodies.

Biostatics, biomedical engineering, bioinformatics, computational biology, and high-level business management are, some of the evolving cores of discipline and can be feasibly, an engine for future growth.

To avoid being labeled as cargo cult statistics, these core disciplines need to be included in some form, both at graduate and undergraduate levels, though I was spared of it, in my medical course of the last century.

Internet

Technology became the boon, leaving all the service media behind, becoming almost indispensible, during the Covid-19 of, year 2020. **Health information technology** improved overnight, rather than gradual entry as planned before. Tele-psychiatry was introduced in 1970s, and is now in its advanced mode of video conferencing. Australia, a widespread country with its geographical diversity, is well suited to address its workforce shortage, in the areas of remote, rural, child and adolescent services, by the use of technology. Since 2004 it has steadily grown, as a credible alternative, to the traditional means of face-to-face patient care. Its convincing utility and acceptance has ensured, its future, as a way of life.

Technology is now on the forefront of impressive progress, unraveling the enigma of major psychiatric illnesses, and translating it into clinical utility. Similar to other branches of medicine, psychiatry will also benefit from diagnostic technology, in revealing the brain functions, and developing more reliable, safe and quicker onset drugs, without the potential for abuse.

Online anxiety treatment has gained acceptance, with sizeable recovery and convenience.

Mind Spot, online digital mental health service, is gaining its grounds since 2013.

Although digitalization is claiming to change the long waiting lists, as an outdated idea of twentieth century, by providing right therapy, for right person, at right time with online resources, it may still face its usual challenges of landing on the ground.

Australians generally embrace technology fairly promptly. The most popular doctor in the world "Dr Google MD", can no longer be overlooked. Most of the households have **Internet connections**, and nearly 90% own a smart phone (Deloitte Australia.2018). Widespread Internet access has changed, health-seeking behavior. 80% Australians, report searching, the Internet for health information. Nearly 40% seek health advice on line (Lipton D, et al. 2015).

An Australian study has found, that 34% people attending emergency department, had searched the Internet for information, about their condition (Cocco AM, et al. 2018). There is a saying, 'if you can't beat them, join them'. So, the psychiatrist must acknowledge it, using it for a therapeutic alliance, and it may even be helpful, in joint decision-making. Ask the patient what they have read online, about the condition and its treatment. Providing them with reliable websites may also be useful. It is also likely that the patient may want to discuss the information, acquired online with their psychiatrist.

Diagnostic Applications

One of the developing **tools of digital health technology** is **Symptom Checker**. It is a web based or a smart phone diagnostic app, using artificial intelligence methods, which can provide diagnosis, on the basis of a set of self reported symptoms. It suggests diagnosis on broad range of conditions, and triage advice. Diagnostic apps are, routinely used by medical students, to support their education.

Symptom checker will require further refinement to replace the traditional diagnostic process. An Australian study for its relevance and reliability, rated it as providing 36% correct first diagnosis and appropriate triage advice of 49%.

A wearable sensor **Accelerometer,** detects and monitors the development of movement disorders, like drug induced Parkinsonism. It utilises electronic sensors, to measure linear acceleration forces, of a body part, in 3 orthogonal directions, capturing the movement of the body part, produced by the action of gravity and muscles.

Accelerometers have been widely used, in investigating movement disorders of Parkinson's disease, Huntington's disease, and strokes. With its excellent, correlation with electromyogram data, it can detect typical Parkinson's tremors with high sensitivity and specificity. It is also positively correlated with, the clinical rating scales demonstrating, the potential capability and reliability in detecting, drug induced Parkinsonism including akathisia. In some studies, it has out-performed the precision of, rating scales. Encouraged by the success of the accelerator, the next stage is planning, a wrist-watch sized device, which will be easier for patients to use (Trisno R, et al. 2020).

There has been a revolution in the use of mobile health devices, for monitoring physical health, which is now extending to mental health. Mobile health devices can reliably record biometric data including electro-dermal activity (a measure of perspiration), actigraphy (measuring changes in emotional state), heart-rate and body temperature. As the result of it, possibility of predicting and pre-empting a relapse may not be far. Physiological indicators of stress can provide valuable insights into the unwell mind. The sensors from wearable health devices and mobile phone data predicted high versus low academic performance, sleep quality, mental health and perceived stress with 67-92% accuracy (Sano A 2018).

Online education introduces significant opportunities to enhance educational outcome. With the exponential growth of online resources, virtual classrooms may soon replace, didactic lectures. RANZCP is not far behind in incorporating online educational technology. As the older generation of teachers hesitant in using the full potential of technology, are being replaced by, the younger generation with fluent computer literacy, online learning will become the norm. Nevertheless the nuances of feelings, emotions, modeling and empathy will remain a challenge without personal contact and direct observation.

English author Aldous Huxley in 1932 wrote a dystopian social science fiction novel Brave New World: 5th of the 100 best English language books of 20th century. He envisaged huge scientific advancements in reproductive technology and psychological manipulation. What a fantasy and forecast: I thought to myself, when I read about a Chinese genome company, offering new options in the quest of producing quality children. The new technology will enable social engineering with human embryo not only in detecting an array of genetic conditions, solving some of the social and medical issues but to design a baby of you choice.

If the threat of the takeover by technology wasn't enough for me, I felt even more ancient, reading about the impact of artificial intelligence and machine learning in the field of psychiatry. The computer takes information from the patient and learns from that, identifies the pattern and then makes the decision. I grew up believing that human interactions, subtle emotions, empathy and compassion are totally under the ownership of human beings. Am I prepared to navigate the technological changes in the delivery of patient care? Am I underestimating the pace of technological advances? Will the future generation of psychiatric patients be sitting next to the robot? And what about the safety and ethical concerns? These questions have clouded my mind so much, that I cannot look in to the future, of the collaborative and engaging role of humans and machines, in making high-risk clinical decisions (Cearns M, et al. 2020).

References

Cearns M, Hahn, et al. Machine learning probability calibration of high-risk clinical decision-making ANZJP 2020. Vol 54 (2) 123-126.

Cocco AM, Zordon R et al. Dr Google in ED: searching for online health information by adult emergency department patients. Med J Aust. 2018: 209: 342-347.

Deloitte Australia mobile consumer survey 2018. http://images.content. deloitte.com.au.

Lipton D, Jutal A. "Its like having a physician in your pocket" A critical analysis of self-diagnosis smartphone apps. Soc Sci Med 2015; 133: 128-135.

Sano A, Taylor S, et al. (2018) Identifying objective physiological markers and modifiable behaviours for self reported stress and mental health status using wearable sensors and mobile phones: Observational study. Journal of Medical Internet Research 20: 1-20.

Tranquillity Denied Stress and its Impact today. Anthony Hordern 1976.

Trisno R, Nair P et al. Using accelerometer as a diagnostic tool to detect drug induced Parkinsonism secondary to first generation anti psychotic medications. Australasian Psychiatry 2020 28(3) 348-353.

CIRCADIAN SCIENCE

THE EVOLUTION OF circadian science, involving coordination of environment and internal biological clock (supra-chiasmatic nucleus SCN), has been a remarkable step, in uncovering the mind brain dualism, and the mystery of body's response across multiple time zones. The term circadian comes from the Latin phrase circa *diem* (around a day). 24 hours cycles that are, part of body's internal clock, running in the background, to carry out essential functions and processes.

Circadian rhythm exists, in most of the organisms. For example it helps flowers, open and close at night at the right times, and plants have seasonal rather than 24 hours cycle. It keeps nocturnal animals, from leaving their shelter, during the daytime, when they will be exposed to more predators

Circadian rhythm has been a significant inclusion, in the progress of psychiatry, and has been instrumental in developing new medications. It has also helped in understanding the environmental impact, on mental states. The synchronisation of circadian rhythm, and the biological (master) clock, with help of light, regulates multiple body functions. One of the most important circadian rhythm is sleep wake cycle.

Pineal gland, also known as master gland is light sensitive and is connected to the biological clock SCN.

During the day, light exposure causes the master clock to send signals, which generates alertness and helps us keep awake and active.

At night master clock initiates the production of melotonin a sleep-promoting hormone, by the pineal body, regulating sleep-wake cycle. Pineal body also secretes serotonin during the daylight.

Melotonin is a powerful antioxidant as well, with its impact on growth hormone and release of sex hormones. It plays vital role in regulating metabolism, growth and reproduction

When properly aligned, a circadian rhythm can promote consistent and restorative sleep. It is a significant pathway in the development and course of various illnesses like the link between sleep and bipolar disorder. Sleep disruption in bipolar disorder may be due to a weaker coupling of the circadian system to external environment (Harvey2008).

It can also play integral role in diverse aspects of physical and mental systems. The digestive system produces protein to match the typical times of the meals and the endocrine system regulates the hormones to suit normal energy expenditure.

SCN is highly sensitive to light, which serves as the critical external clue that, influences the signals it sends, to coordinate the internal clock. Although exercise, social activities and temperature can affect the master clock, light is the most powerful influence on circadian rhythm.

Circadian rhythm plays role in regulation of blood sugar, cholesterol, immune system as well as process of DNA repair: involved in preventing cancer. It can influence the effectiveness of anticancer drugs. Circadian rhythm can be a risk factor for mental illness as well, like depression, bipolar disorder and potential for neurodegenerative diseases like dementia (Brainard J, et al. 2015).

A subtype of recurrent depression, a rapidly evolving area: seasonal affective disorder (SAD) is caused by decreased environmental light in winter, which is a pathological variant of, commonly experienced low mood, in darker than, lighter months. It has high frequency of 15% of mania and 25% of depressive bipolar episodes

Although it responds to artificial bright light, is no better than either antidepressant medication or CBT. There remains scepticism about the SAD construct (Murray 2017) and its putative association with poor outcome (Geoffroy 2014).

It also affects the so-called jetlag when varying and increasing number of time zones are crossed within a short period of time. Until the person's circadian rhythm can acclimatise to the day night cycle of the new location, they are likely to suffer from sleeping problems and fatigue.

Shift work disorder is widely recognised as disrupting the circadian rhythm.

There are, simple measure to overcome, the sleep impairment. Exposure to natural light specially, early in the day helps reinforce the strongest circadian clue. Artificial light exposure at night and electronic devices leading up to bedtime can interfere with circadian rhythm.

There is some evidence that light intensity higher than 500-lux, suppresses melotonin secretion, which may be a risk factor for mood episodes. Social Rhythm Therapy including sleep and circadian regulation, focusing on regular daily rhythm in relation to sleep and wake time, meal times and socialisation, provides a potentially useful model for inpatient therapy. It involves regular time to wake up for the benefit of exposure to daylight, which is crucial for re-establishing circadian rhythm as light is the primary synchronising agent. Food is required to initiate the rhythm for hormone release activated by the peripheral clock in the liver. This peripheral clock helps to synchronise the day and night cycle of SCN. Social clues entrain the circadian rhythm to form a link between biological and psychological processes (Wirz-JusticeA, et al 2013).

Reference

Brainard J, Gobel M et al. 2015. Health implications of disrupted circadian rhythm and the potential for daylight saving, as therapy. Anaesthesiology 122 (5), 1170-1175.

Geoffroy PA, Bellivier F, et al. Seasonality and bipolar disorder: A systematic review, from admission rates to seasonality of symptoms. Journal of Affective Disorders 168:210-223.

Harvey A (2008) Sleep and circadian rhythm in bipolar disorder: Seeking synchrony, harmony and regulation. American Journal of Psychiatry 165: 820-829.

Murray G SAD schmad: Is seasonal affective disorder a valid construct? ANZJP 2017 Vol 51(!) 18-19.

Wirz-Justice A Benedetti F, et al. (2013) Chronotherapeutics For Affective Disorders: A Clinician Manual for Light and Wake Therapy.: Karger.

ECO SYSTEM

"We have not inherited the environment but have
borrowed it from our future generations"

ECOSYSTEM IS DEFINED as a geographical area, where plants, animals and other organisms, as well as weather, and landscape, work together to form a bubble of life. It is the basic unit of the field of scientific study of nature, made up of 2 inseparable components.

Biotic: Set of living organism such as animal, plants and micro organisms that are in constant interaction and interdependent.

Abiotic: specific physical environment such as climate, temperature, humidity, concentration of nutrients and ph.

The concept of soma-terratic and psycho terratic were introduced, at the 2006 RANZCP conference in Cairns 'Creating Future', predicting the effect of contaminated ecosystem on mind and body. It was well illustrated with the raging bushfires across the country with warnings, in no uncertain terms, of serious health consequences. Mental health cannot be spared, either as the direct result of, or secondary to physical illnesses caused by the environmental contamination.

Environmentally sustainable health care system is now on the agenda of priorities. Over the past few decades, world attention has shifted from communicable to non-communicable diseases, which is reversing with the unprecedented pandemic virus Covid-19.

Due its profound impact on every aspect of life in every country and environment, the future cannot be fully projected: the kind of mental disorder it may generate (Madden D, 2020).

Mental health consequences of disasters can persist for many years after the event, related to physical, social and individual changes. Nevertheless all large studies of disaster survivors converge on the observation, that most people are resilient, and do not develop psychiatric disorders (Norris FH, et al. 2009).

Climate Change

Climate Change is likely to be a collage of unfolding disasters with uncertain consequences. There are predictions of temperature rises in the future with possibilities of extreme temperature and heat waves. Already there is evidence around the world of the devastation it may cause. Victorian heat wave review (Department of Health and Human services Victorian government 2009) concluded 'the elderly and very elderly have been found ... specially, at risk'. Deaths directly related to heat; heatstroke, hyperthermia and dehydration increased massively. It was far worse for people with mental illness and those taking psychotropic medications.

International, Intergovernmental Panel on Climate Change, an authoritative panel of 1250 experts, approved by 194 governments is emphatic: warming of the climate system is unequivocal. In their 2014 report they have forecasted that Australia may face disproportionate risks of temperature increases outpacing global warming worldwide, heat waves becoming more frequent, intense and longer with increasing risk of drought and desertification (Intergovernmental Panel on Climate Change).

Extreme weather events increase acute traumatic stress disorder, post-traumatic stress disorder, depression, anxiety, substance use and stress related relationship disharmony. Indirect effects will arise primarily from damage to land, infrastructure and community functioning, leading to climate related migration. In a large Australian epidemiological study average monthly temperature increases, were associated with significant rise in suicide rate (Qi X, et al. 2015).

In 2014, WHO held its first dedicated conference on climate change and health, concluding that climate change will have, the defining issue for the health systems, in 21st century. Health professionals have the knowledge, cultural authority and responsibility to protect health from climate change.

Medical profession has responsibility to provide clear and compelling examples of, health consequences of climate disruption.

Mental health professionals specially, clinicians need to be mindful, of reducing carbon footprints of our institutions, practices and other activities. Reducing waste in clinical care, avoiding unnecessary tests, minimising nonattendance, promoting early intervention and integrating, models of care, remains our responsibility (Maugham DL, et al 2015).

References

Core Writing Team RK Pachauri and LA Myer (eds) Geneva: IPPC. Intergovernmental Panel on Climate Change (IPCC) (2014) Climate Change 2014: Synthesis Report. Contribution of Working Groups 1,2 and 3 to the Fifth Assessment Report of the Intergovernmental Panel on Climate Change. Core Writing Team.

Madden D, Capon A, Truskett P Environmentally sustainable health care: now is time for action, MJA 2012 (8). 4May 2020.

Maugham DL and Davidson P 2015. Need for sustainable psychiatry. The Lancet Psychiatry 2: 675-677.

Norris FH, Tracey M, et al. (2009) Looking for resilience: understanding the longitudinal trajectory of responses to stress. Social Science and Medicine 68: 2190-2198.

Qi X, Hu W, et al. 2015 Associations between climate variability, unemployment, and suicide in Australia: A multicity study BMC Psychiatry15: 114.

SPIRITUALITY AND PSYCHIATRY

A calm mind is not just peaceful; it is
focused, self directing and divine"

SPIRITUALITY; STILL REMAINS a nebulous concept for an average person, difficult to define. However to pin it in words, it can be defined as the quest for meaning and purpose in life, with pursuits of truth and values in the search of transcendence. It is a personal experience, whilst religion is a community centered ritual, and events in relationship to God.

Religion has been a taboo subject in science and medicine, despite mounting evidence that it helps in understanding and in accepting the adverse situations like illness. It increases the rapport between the patient and the therapist with possible link of commonality, and start of a grip on patient's personal life.

Australians and New Zealanders are, less religious than the society in the US, though with the influx of immigrants, it is likely to change. One study found spiritual growth is important to some 70% of US adults, so situating mindfulness training in a spiritual frame may be culturally congruent for a significant proportion of Western population.

There are continuing studies comprehensively documenting the positive effect of religiousness on physical and mental health (Koenig HG,

2012). There is strong evidence that increased sense of spirituality is one mechanism of mindfulness based stress reduction benefit for wellbeing.

Religion is unlikely to vanish. It continues to be important for significant number of older adults.

The role of religion and spirituality in mortality, coping and recovery has been well documented. Patients often express, desire to discuss spirituality with their doctors. They want their doctor to be aware of their religious and spiritual beliefs (McLean CD, et al. 2003).

I have often wondered about the resemblance between psychotherapy, psychoanalysis, spirituality and Indian philosophy. Having come from a background where culturally engrained spirituality was the unspoken ingredient of raising a child, mastering one's mind was life long desired pursuit and failing it; was seen as the character weakness, I do endorse spirituality. This helps in grooming a well-integrated and resourceful person with resilience, ability to compromise, empathy and acceptance of inevitability of death. Spirituality not only contributes to healing but also towards finding meaning in suffering and acceptance of the illness.

As much as I valued the role of psychotherapy/ analysis uncovering the inner feelings, be it spiritual or otherwise, in comprehensive patient management, I felt ill at ease in becoming a full time psychotherapist. Well, to learn more about it to dispel my ignorance, I did enroll in a training program, which required self-therapy/analysis first. Although I enjoyed the focused attention on the couch with an attentive listener for an hour, a rare event in real life, I did not feel I could go on for months. So I was contented to making my life, just as a psychiatrist, which I found more stimulating.

Closing this chapter, without highlighting the long neglected unlimited potential of spiritual science, emanating from the country of my birth, will not only be ignorant but will show the fragility of my convictions. Meditation and Yoga practices and other experiments of spirituality are increasingly recognized in rousing willpower and mental strength along with sharpening of intellect. Self-control through spiritual wakening may be able to explain the difference between the powerful and powerless man.

Many people, from all walks of life, over many centuries, allover the world, have shown the supernatural and spiritual powers defying the common beliefs and even the laws of the nature. Meditation practices, in many of its forms may be the discerning factor between the mind control and determination of people with supernatural powers and the people with feeble mentality. It may allow a healthy mind to live in an unhealthy body.

The author of 2,700 books and translator of the entire Vedic Vangmaya Pandit Shree Ram Sharma Acharya received bare formal education. He pioneered the revival of spirituality and creative integration of the modern and ancient sciences and religion. He became a legend in his own lifetime. (Human Brain).

The unexplained enigma remains about the remarkable contributions made by the eminent scientist Stephen Hawking in unraveling the secrets, of the cosmos. Diagnosed with a deadly disease early in his life which paralyzed all of his four limbs eventually losing his voice., he was regarded as the second Einstein of the last century. A great mathematician and astrophysicist, he was the distinguished professor the Cambridge University.

The only university, for handicapped people in the world, was established in India by the Jagadguru Rambhadracharya. in 2001. Jagadguru was blind from the age of 2 months and had no formal education till the age of 17 years. He never used any aid to learn or compose including Braille. He can speak 22 languages, is a spontaneous poet and writer in several languages including Sanskrit. He has authored more than 100 books and over 50 papers. He is regarded as one of the greatest authorities on Ramayan and is its Critical Editor.

So how do we explain the outstanding super human accomplishments of these people?

There is a huge unexplored field of human brain potential, evidenced by people's experiences and abilities, beyond the scope of this book.

Only about 7% of the powers of intellectual and scholarly brain, are used. 93% of the capabilities of human brain weighing only about 3 pounds, still remain unused. Creating its replica through artificial intelligence may not be possible, due to the natural propensity for its growth and re-growth, and its functioning in toto.

ETHICS IN SYCHIATRY

ETHICS IS DESCRIBED as the moral value, honesty and respect in treating our patients, which is very similar to professionalism underpinning the trust the public has in doctors. It ensures that we practice safely with dignity and are accountable. It involves informed consent, confidentiality, maintaining trust in doctor patient relationship, showing awareness of their limitations, demonstrating health and probity, life-long learning and understanding the relevance of outside bodies (RCP). However our autonomy is just as important as the moral obligation to respect our patients' autonomy. According to Hippocratic oath we must have best and selfless intention to benefit the patient with our knowledge and experience, minimising any possibility of deliberate harm. Empowerment of the patient must also be aimed as part of the treatment. Patients' equality and rights must be respected though within the context of prevailing rules and regulations of the organisation/country.

Psychiatrists have always been ethically obligated, to uphold the integrity of the medical profession overall, by expressing their views in a way that avoids, self-promotion or denigration of others. In order to promote the integrity of psychiatric profession, ethically driven clinical practice serving the best interest of the patients must remain the highest priority.

The role of pharmaceutical industry has been debated fiercely since the outset of this century and gradually became an ethical issue. International conferences: a hub for psychiatrists to pick up on trends, networking, and learn new things, became heavily subsidised market place, for the pharmaceutical industries. As much as we need them, there was disquiet about the impact of their marketing, and commercial interference on our prescribing. When people holding positions of responsibility are motivated to act in ways opposed to the primary purpose of their position, conflict of interest arises.

There has been strong emphasis laid on prescribing, for rational consideration of the cost and benefit to the patient, based on scientific evidence and objective view. Although the advertisements, which apear in medical journals, are appraised for its authenticity, the detailed appraisal may not be possible.

References

Human Brain Apparent Boon of the Omnipotent by Pandit Shriram Sharma Acharya

Koenig HG, McCullough, Carson D B. Handbook of Religion and Health 2nded. New York: Oxford University Press2012.

McLean CD, Susi B, Phifer N, et al. patient preference for physician discussion and practice of spirituality: results from multi centre patient survey. J Gen Intern med 2003; 18: 38-43.

RCP A competency based curriculum for specialist core training in psychiatry. htpp://www.rcpsych.ac.uk/pdf/CORE CURRICULUM 2010 MAR 2012.pdf.update

PHYSICAL HEALTH

THE USE OF organic/psychiatric dichotomy is not only divisive but is the source of discrimination and stigmatisation. Psychiatric disorders are organic with biological correlates like any other medical condition and should be promoted as a credible branch of medicine.

Modifiable health risk behaviours are key contributors to chronic disease, morbidity and mortality, worldwide. Compared to general population, people with mental illness have higher prevalence of the key risk factors: Tobacco, poor diet, alcohol and low level of physical activity (Bartlem K, et al. 2015a). These risky behaviours, influence the development of metabolic risks such as obesity, diabetes and hypertension. The potential contribution of antipsychotic medications cannot be ignored.

Premature mortality is increased among those with severe mental illness, mainly due to premature deaths from chronic physical health conditions (Firth 2019)

The role of nutrition in health cannot be overemphasized. Knowledge of the importance of nutrition on health is said to go back to nearly 3000 years. Every neurotransmitter goes through many metabolic steps to ensure its synthesis, uptake and breakdown. Every step requires enzymes and every enzyme is dependent upon multiple coenzymes. A variety of minerals and vitamins are required as coenzymes in most of these steps.

Slow acceptance of nutritional intervention is not unusual. Captain James Lancaster carried out a cohort study in 1601, which showed that lemon juice prevented scurvy. In a voyage from England to India, sailors on one ship took daily lemon juice and on the other three ships did not. Halfway through the voyage none of the lemon juice group died, whilst 40% of the sailors in the other ships perished. The experiment was repeated in 1747, by James Lind a physician. Despite evidence the practice did not change. It took another 48 years for the British navy to order citrus fruits for the navy ships. However the universal preventive policy was not enacted for another 70 years when British Board of Trade adopted the innovation. So it took 264 years for the change in national policy (Berwick 2003).

The second Australian survey of psychosis in 2010 revealed that more than half of 4189 participants met the criteria of metabolic syndrome: substantial risk for cardiovascular disease, ¾ were overweight or obese, 9 out of 10 women had abdominal obesity and almost half were hypertensive. Most of them lived on deficient diet and minimal exercise.

Late life depression affects 2-5% elderly patients and is associated with cerebrovascular comorbidity with bilateral risk. It can account for up to 50% late life depression. Depression in all ages increases the risk of venous thrombus embolism. Micro-emboli accumulate gradually over the years impacting on global brain function with cognitive decline and depression.

Physical health monitoring and support, screening and lifestyle interventions, and integrated care pathways are, some of the recommendations put forward by RANZCP, to improve physical health and life expectancy of people with mental illness. The evidence suggests that at least 30% of all people with a long-term physical condition also have a mental health problem. It has also been estimated that 46% people, with mental health problems, have a long-term physical condition (Naylor C, et al. 2012 London). The causal relationship is likely to be bi-directional.

The trajectory of compromised physical health begins rapidly within the first 12 weeks of commencing psychotropic medication. Structured lifestyle interventions from the outset of the treatment like smoking, physical activity; nutrition and weight gain can attenuate medication emergent adverse effects.

The importance of mental health, for physical health cannot be overemphasized.

Physical and psychiatric co and multi-morbidity are common for many obvious reasons, within and beyond the control of the patient.

It is also associated with reciprocally poorer psychiatric and medical outcomes (Penninx BW.2017).

Patients with mental illness, can experience long delays in the diagnosis, of physical illness for a variety of reasons, including the phenomenon known as Diagnostic Overshadowing: the misattribution of physical symptoms to mental illness or its treatment. Therefore it is important to exclude organic illness in patients who present with atypical symptoms, even in the context of long standing psychiatric illness.

A large, WHO study found that co existence of mental and physical ill health was associated with 17-46% increase in health cost. The prevalence of major depressive illness is almost double in medically ill people. Neurological disorders are strongly linked with increased rates of major depressive disorders, with estimated lifetime prevalence, of 20-40% across stroke, epilepsy, multiple sclerosis, traumatic brain injury, Alzheimer's disease and Parkinson's disease (Bhattarai. N, et al. 2013). Other common co-morbid disorders with high risk; include cancer, cerebrovascular diseases, HIV and chronic obstructive pulmonary disease.

Both pharmacological and psychosocial treatments are, recommended though with awareness of possible liver and renal impairment, as well as drug interactions.

Wellness clinic model has been trialed for hard to engage patients within mental health service settings, with positive outcome of better health and cost saving (Stanley SH, et al. 2020).

Mindfulness interventions are equally effective for depression, anxiety as well as for physical symptoms of long-term medical conditions. Mindfulness can be described as bringing one's complete attention to the experiences occurring in the present moment in a non-judgemental, and accepting way (Ludwig DS, et al. 2008). It is a form of meditation practice, which can help cope with pain and disability by altering biological pathways like immune system, autonomic nervous system and neuroendocrine functions. Mindfulness based stress reduction, reduces stress-evoked cortisol level and post-stress inflammatory response.

At the time of writing this book, the world was under the siege, with the unrelenting grip of Covid-19, over the preceding 12 months: considered to be the most transforming event in the last 100 years. As mental health is the first one, to take the brunt of any life adversity, there are predictions of its long-term serious implications on human life. It is far worse for mentally ill people who rely on the support and care of the higher functioning family and community members and have elevated risk of relapse. As the Covid 19 has created anxiety and uncertainty amongst all levels of people, the support network cannot be available as before. Our patients have reduced immunity, a risk factor for contracting the virus, and decompensating or exacerbating their illness. Undue hyper-vigilance leads to stress, and may affect the sleep cycle, compromising the immune system. Impact of social isolation on depression, cannot be ignored.

Covid-19 is the most unusual, unprecedented experience, which cannot be justified as a disaster due to its enduring and unknown trajectory and its global-spread. Nevertheless it is a potential risk factor for PTSD. After nearly 12 months there is no respite, negatively impacting on damage control and damage assessment. It will have implications for any prospective research or longitudinal study due to people's reluctance to get involved, their changed circumstances and most of it, the time lapse. There are many risk factors, for the onset of PTSD and even more moderators, for adaption, in the months and years after trauma exposure (Brewin et al 2000). So how accurately the research will be able to reflect on the health consequences of Covid-19: only time will tell.

The entire social structure has changed with Covid-19 pandemic, undermining the performance of high functioning people as well. The psychiatric sequel may slowly progress for many years, to make deep-seated negative changes in health and personality. One third of 90 survivors of the SARS outbreak in Hong Kong in 2003 had psychiatric disorder 30 months post SARS most commonly PTSD and depression (Mak IW, et al.).

CONSULTATION-LIAISON

CONSULTATION LIAISON PSYCHIATRY: Has been defined as, the interface between general medicine and psychiatry an area of clinical psychiatry which includes all diagnostic, therapeutic, teaching and research activities of psychiatrists in the non psychiatric part of general hospital (Lipowski ZL).

The earliest record of general hospital psychiatry was in 1728 when a mentally ill patient was admitted to Guy's hospital in London. As a profession it was developed in 1930s and appears to have been pioneered with research grant from then Rockefeller Foundation to stimulate collaboration between physicians and psychiatrists.

So it is not a new discipline; to focus on multi morbidity needs, though has suffered from long overdue support and acceptance from both physical and psychiatric health experts.

Prevalence estimates of psychiatric disorders among the medically ill in general hospitals vary between 20 to 40%. However the mean rates of referrals are only 1 to 4% (Ellen S, et al.2006).

The commonest referrals are, for depression, borderline personality disorder, suicide-risk, past psychiatric history, organic mental disorder, substance abuse, and psychosis.

A Case Study

A 51 years old mother of 2 children was referred to CL psychiatry where I was doing my rotation term. She was, brought to hospital emergency, by her family, with her bleeding amputated hand, wrapped in a towel. Mrs L was, found by her family, sitting in the bathroom using the saw to cut through her non-dominant wrist. She was admitted to plastic surgery ward. Her hand was reattached though with partially lost functions.

She lost her husband a month earlier with whom she lived in emotionally fulfilling relationship since the age of 19 years. There was no previous or family history of any mental health issue. She was working as a schoolteacher at the time. Her husband's death was sudden at the peak of their married life when they were preparing for a lifelong dream of a well earned, 6 months holiday.

She spoke very little, slept poorly and ate sparingly following the death, remaining in the company of her family.

On examination she was monosyllable though co-operative and said that she felt no pain and was dissociated from the bleeding.

She was transferred to the psychiatric unit after 10 days when she stabilised from her surgery. She required close observation due to her seemingly depressed mood, and violent nature of her self-injury. She remained, hospitalised, for 6 weeks, was treated with antidepressants having declined ECT. Her diagnosis was pathological grief. She made steady progress though not to her premorbid level which was not surprising considering what the loss meant for her. She was planning to return to work in due course. She was closely followed up by the community mental health team and continued on medication.

Major self-mutilations are rare, majority are men and mostly as the result of psychosis and are unlikely to have previous history of serious self-injury. In the presenting case the mutilation may have resulted from the internal turmoil. In many cultures around the world, suicide after husband's death is considered honourable.

She suffered from prolonged/complex grief disorder. The syndrome is characterised by intense yearning for the deceased, distress at the lost relationship, disbelief, difficulty with acceptance, avoidance of reminders, a sense that life became meaningless and purposeless, self-identity confusion, emotional numbness, bitterness, loss of trust and difficulty in re-engaging with life, which goes on for more than 6 months with functional impairment (Maercker A, et al. 2013).

While some people experience enduring, disabling levels of distress, many experience symptoms that gradually decline with little or no disruption in functioning, following bereavement.

A serious self-injury like the aforementioned patient, require multidisciplinary approach. Prompt CL psychiatric care improves both surgical and psychiatric outcome. Collaboration of surgical and psychiatric team is essential. CL psychiatrist has a clear role supporting staff and managing countertransference. Family may also require counseling and understanding of the situation.

CL psychiatry in general hospitals is cost effective, and when involved early in admission, it may reduce length of stay. With regular support and mental health training of acute hospital staff, it provides comprehensive and high quality service both for the patient and the family.

Consultation liaison team may be required to manage acutely and severely disturbed patients in casualty, like intoxicated and head injury requiring, prudent and quick management. General principles to be observed are avoiding poly-pharmacy, or synergistic effects of certain drugs in suppressing respiration or causing arrhythmia. Benzodiazepines should be cautiously used.

The most effective IM medications in reducing agitation are: droperidole, haloperidol and lorazepam, which can also be sedating. Fast acting IV drugs include midazolam, lorazepam, dro and haloperidol. Combination of IM haloperidol and promethazine or olanzapine, have been shown to have superior control (Innes J et al. 2013).

Psychosomatic Illnesses: "The sorrow which has no vent in tears may make other organs weep".

Somatisation disorder once referred to as hysteria, to express psychological distress by physical symptoms, can be traced back to pre Hippocratic Egyptians Psychosomatic Illnesses involves both mind and body with bidirectional impact. It is now well established that brain, mind and body have reciprocal relationship. Correlation of functional gastrointestinal disorders, as well as many other physical illnesses, with anxiety and depression is the expected comorbidity.

Anxiety and depression increases sympathetic and decreases parasympathetic tone in the autonomic nervous system and impacts on hypothalamic pituitary Adrenal axis (HPA), resulting in raised levels of cortisol and corticotrophin releasing factor (Messay B, et al. 2012). These complex and self-perpetuating effects alter the ecology of gut lumen flora, increasing motility, secretion and sensitivity, which is seen in irritable bowel syndrome, making it more susceptible to systemic inflammation with exposure to gut bacteria.

The gut inflammation in response to E coli leads to excessive tumour necrosis factor alpha, which causes anxiety and depression (Collins SM, et al. 2012).

Psychological distress and gastrointestinal symptoms, are often found sequentially in the same patient.

Separation of children between the ages of 5 and 18 years is associated with IBS and parental divorce over 18 months was associated with functional dyspepsia (Koloski AK, et al.18).

Chronic pain is one of the commonest and complex psychosomatic symptoms associated with significant psychiatric morbidity: a burden not only to the patient but also to the health care system. Developmental factors such as adverse childhood experiences, insecure attachment and dysfunctional emotional processing may predispose individuals to chronic pain (Lane 2018).

References

Bartlem K, Bowman J, et al. (2015a) Chronic disease health risk behaviours amongst people with mental illness. ANZJP 49: 731-741.

Berwick DM (2003) Disseminating innovations in health care. Journal of the American Medical Association 289: 1969-1975.

Bhattarai. N, Charlton J, Rudisil C et al. 2013 prevalence of depression and utilisation of health care in single and multiple morbidity: A population based cohort study Psychological Medicine 43: 1423-1431.

Brewin CR, Andrews B, et-al. (2000) Meta-analysis of risk factors for post-traumatic stress disorder in trauma-exposed adults. Journal of Consulting and Clinical Psychology 68: 748-766.

Collins SM, Surette M, et al. 2012 Interplay between intestinal micro biota and brain. Nature Reviews Microbiology 10: 735-742.

Ellen S, Lacey C, Data collection in consultation Liaison psychiatry: an evaluation of Case-mix. Australasian Psychiatry. 2006; 14: 43-45.

Firth J, Siddiqi N, et al. 2019 The Lancet Psychiatry Commission: A blue print for protecting physical health of people with mental illness The Lancet Psychiatry 6: 675-712.

Innes J and Sethi F. Current rapid tranquillization documents in UK: a review of the drugs recommended, their routes of administration and clinical parameters influencing their use. J Psychiatr Intens Care 2013; 9: 110-118.

Koloski AK, Boyce PM, et al. Somatisation an independent psychosocial risk factor for irritable bowel syndrome but not dyspepsia: a population based study European Journal of Gastroenterology and Hepatology 18: 1101-1109.

Lane RD, Anderson FS, et al. Biased competition favouring physical over emotional pain: a possible explanation for the link between early adversity and chronic pain. Psychosom Med 2018; 80: 880-890.

Lipowski ZL. Psychosomatic Medicine and Liaison Psychiatry: Selected Papers. New York: Plenum Medical Book Company.

Ludwig DS, Kabat-Zin J. 2008 Mindfulness in medicine. Journal of the American Medical Association 300:1350-1352.

Maercker A, Brewin CR, et al. 2013 Proposals for mental disorders specifically associated with stress in the International Classification of Diseases 11. The Lancet 381: 1683-1685.

Mak IW, Chu CM, et al. Long-term psychiatric morbidities among SARS survivors. General Hospital Psychiatry 31:318-326.

Messay B, Lim A, et al. 2012 Current understanding of the bidirectional relationship of major depression with inflammation. Biology of Mood and Anxiety disorder 2:1-4.

Naylor C, Pasonage M, et al. 2012 Long-term conditions and mental health. London: The King's Fund.

Penninx BW.2017. Depression and cardiovascular disease: epidemiological evidence on their linking mechanism. Neuroscience and Bio-behavioural Reviews 74: 277-286.

Stanley SH, Velayudhan A, et al. Physical health wellness clinic model of care for patients with mental health issues who are hard to engage. Australasian Psychiatry. 2020 Vol 28 (3) 303-306.

DIAGNOSIS IN PSYCHIATRY

EMIL KRAEPELIN, THE father of descriptive psychiatry left us with 2 major disorders manic-depressive psychosis and dementia praecox, now we have 18 categories of illnesses.

There are genuine concerns expressed, that boundaries of illnesses will broaden, because of changes in DSM-5, resulting in medicalization of, range of normal behaviour more than the earlier editions: open to exploitation. The professional drift of psychiatry, to drag normal human experiences into realm of psychopathology, has resulted in diagnostic inflation, with ever-growing assortments of classification of, questionable clinical and research validity, culminating in DSM-5 (Frances 2014).

It is interesting to note the impact of mental health literacy with easy access to diagnostic manuals, which has allowed people, outside mental health professionals, to become diagnosticians with no underlying knowledge of the illness. Psychiatric jargon and self-diagnosis is becoming almost a common usage.

There are 2 major sources to classify psychiatric illnesses ICD International Classification of Diseases by World Health Organisation and DSM Diagnostic and Statistical Manual of Mental Health by American Psychiatric Association.

Both of these are regularly updated to refine the diagnosis for its best treatment. Nevertheless psychiatry is still rated, as not doing well according to United Nations Authority (Special Rapporteur human rights Council 2017).

The concern that neither DSM nor ICD represent valid disease entity, as their criteria and categories were formulated before our current knowledge of neuroscience, and perhaps do not reflect the organisation of brain circuits and their associated behaviours: the U.S National Institute of Mental Health has developed Research Domain Criteria (RDoC). It has long term goals of developing a biologically based classification system, beginning, by looking at specific neurobiological or behavioural domain, or constructs like anxiety, attention and working memory via various units of analysis (genetic, molecular, physiological and behavioural) regardless of DSM 5 or ICD 11 diagnostic category.

RDoC does not try to define a cut-off between normal and abnormal, instead, examining the dimensional trajectory between normal and disturbed (Francis A. 2014.). RDoC encourages a new research framework on mental disorder. It can define meaningful subgroups for the purpose of pathophysiological studies and treatment selection and provide pathways by which research findings can be translated into changes in clinical decision-making (Morris SB, et al. 2012).

Schizophrenia is much less prominent in DSM-5 than in DSM-4. It stresses that people with symptoms and sign of psychosis, should be evaluated on all core domains like delusions, hallucinations, abnormal thoughts, behaviour and negative symptoms, with intention of simplifying the diagnosis.

Schizoaffective disorder was first coined in 1933 by Kasanin, as reactive psychosis, which was accepted only after initial ambivalence, by DSM-3 in 1980. It is defined as severe mental health disorder, characterised by both psychotic and mood symptoms either concurrently or at different time points, during the illness. With its clinical and aetiological overlap, major mood episode should be present, for most of the disorder's duration to make the boundary with schizophrenia clear. Structural abnormalities in patients with schizoaffective disorder are widespread across various brain areas. However research supporting a diagnostic category is weak at best, not globally accepted, and it still appears to be an uninvited member of DSM. The loosely defined DSM diagnostic criteria of over the 4 decades, has been of no discernible benefit to patients, and nor indeed the doctors gained any valuable insight (Malhi GS 2013).

There are some differences between DSM-5 and ICD, specially, in diagnosing schizophrenia. Illness duration of 6 months is required in DSM-5 and one month in ICD. DSM-5, proposes dimensional assessment of symptoms and related phenomenon.

DSM diagnoses have much more weight in treatment decisions than ICD: all current pharmacological treatments are based on studies designed around diagnoses from DSM. Our newest diagnostic manuals have created diagnoses for which treatment do not currently exist (Ostacher 2014).

Psychiatry with its ever-increasing domain of including, most human adversities and behaviours, as pathological, has caused grave concerns both within and outside the profession. Mental health disorders are estimated to account for up to one third of global burden of diseases and top 5 contributors to the years of life lost. (Vigo D, et al. 2016).

So, are we over-diagnosing? Possibly. Can we capture the mind to the same extent, as we can explore the brain with advances in neuroscience and technology? This may generate the confusion of over-diagnosis. Presentation of emotional /mental symptoms must be weighed in the context of the events, culture, family and relationships to classify it as normal or pathological.

It was interesting to see that the editor of ANZJP Prof G Malhi created a section in the journal for Fake View Series in July 2019. In an age where everything can be seemingly, fake, Prof Malhi started to examine contentious ideas and concepts in psychiatry in search of truth. It resulted in pruning of overgenerous medicalization of human behaviour. It has also been relevant to the conflicting information, which comes not only through media, but from medical literature as well. As the result of it, the world appears to have adapted to believing, any sensational health related news with a grain of salt, as most evidences seem to be followed by counter evidence. The recent good example was when I read about wheat and milk being unhealthy. These have been the two staple food items, part of my daily diet, and considered essential for good health.

I must share an anecdote which was also confirmed by a study, an experience of mine, questioning the long held view of legitimacy and accuracy of psychiatric diagnoses.

In 1974 when I was a trainee at Callan Park hospital, there was a commotion amongst us, to watch out for the pseudo-patients. Apparently the psychology department, of Sydney University was, sending healthy volunteers pretending with psychotic symptoms who were duly admitted, diagnosed and treated against their will. It is not difficult to imagine the reactions of our profession with the uncovering of the reality of these fake patients.

David Rosenhan, a psychology professor at Stanford University conducted an experiment and published it with the title of 'On being sane in insane places'. Dr Rosehan along with 7 other healthy associates presented to 12 different psychiatric hospitals, all complaining of auditory hallucinations. Once admitted, the pseudo-patients ceased displaying symptoms, and behaved normally. These patients were hospitalised for an average of 19 days with a diagnosis of schizophrenia and discharged with credit of successful treatment. Rosenhan was justified in questioning the validity of psychiatric diagnoses, given that the hospital was not able to separate sane from insane.

In another anecdote one of our consultants used to share, was a disturbed patient with, good command of English brought to hospital by a relative, who had limited language proficiency. The patient was able to convince the admitting doctor that the relative was ill, needing the hospital care. The relative's attempts, to rectify the situation were taken as, aggression and refusal of treatment, which resulted in forced administration of psychotropic drugs, whilst the real patient eloped. Finally the situation was reversed when the police brought the real patient with some family members to the admission center.

Both ICD and DSM rely on subjective clinical acumen in absence of any objective biological markers, which can vary dangerously against the interest of the patient.

References

Francis A. (2014). RDoC is necessary, but very oversold. World Psychiatry.13: 47-49.

Francis A (2014) How many psychiatric diagnoses fit on the head of a pin? ANZJP 48:1067-1068.

Malhi GS. Making up schizoaffective disorder: Cosmetic changes to a sad creation ANZJP 47(10) 891-894.

Morris SB, Cuthbert B N. 2012 Research Domain Criteria: cognitive systems, neural circuits and dimensions of behaviour. Dialogues in Clinical Neuroscience 14: 29-37.

Ostacher M. What can ICD-11be that, DSM 5 cannot? ANZJP 2014. Vol 48 (3) 283-284.

RosenhanDL. On being sane in insane places. Science 1973; 179: 250-258.

Vigo D, Thornicroft G et al. Estimating the true global burden of mental illness. Lancet Psychiatry 2016; 3: 171-178

ACADEMIC PSYCHIATRY AND RESEARCH

CRITICAL AND SCIENTIFIC thinking, continuing education, research, writing and publications are the markers of clinical credibility for the medical profession. With this in mind The Australian Association of Psychiatrists was established in 1946 (a College of colleagues). It was taken over by the Royal Australian New Zealand College of Psychiatrists (RANZCP) in 1963, which was the most significant progress in refining Australian psychiatry and taking it to the world stage. Australasian Psychiatric Quarterly Newsletter the forerunner of ANZJP: was published in1948 by its founder editor and the president of the AAP: Dr Allan Stoller.

RANZCP

RANZCP must be applauded for its continuous endeavour to improve mental health care for all those who need it, by lobbying the government, for funding, as well as the interest of the members. It encourages all the Fellows, to actively participate in College activities, and its cutting edge mental health care. It has 3 networks, representing public sector, private and academic psychiatrists.

Gender balance has been on the active agenda of the College as the younger female fellows outnumber the males and 50% of our patients are females. The progressive legacy of RANZCP more than any other medical college has enabled women to play important role in the field of psychiatry, by its flexible training program which allows, part time training as well as break in the training at some point. It is encouraging that nearly 55% of the trainees and over 40% psychiatrists are women. Nevertheless there is paucity of women in senior leadership positions, despite increasing number of women choosing psychiatry for their post-graduate qualification. Unfortunately there still exists, the gender barrier for women doctors to reach their full potential and thrive in positions of power. The governing capacity of committees strengthens, when the range of leadership style is broadened, for its collective capacity of new and robust ideas.

However, with more than 6000 members RANZCP is highly regarded, and is well managed in serving its members and our patients. Nevertheless one of the challenges for the College is, considerable workforce shortage to cater for the increasing mental health needs of Australian population. Despite the overall increase in the number of medical students, the dearth of psychiatry trainees reflect, diminishing interest of the medical students and junior doctors in this discipline. The speculated reasons appear to be, the perception that psychiatry lacks scientific foundation and effective treatments. In the light of continuing shortage, RANZCP along with Department of Health and Ageing, released a promotional DVD 'Psychiatry: a Better Understanding' in 2008, designed to attract potential trainees to a career in Psychiatry. Although the DVD appeared to improve the understanding of the role of a psychiatrist, and interest of the participants, a large percentage of students felt that the DVD had no effect on their understanding, or interest in this profession (Robertson T, et al. 2009).

A similar promotional film was commissioned by Royal College of psychiatrist (R C Psych) in 2013 'A Different Life' replicating the findings of RANZCP DVD.

The Claassen Institute of psychiatry at the University of Western Australia was established in 2008 as an enrichment program for medical students. A week-long program enables the students to gain a range of different perspectives of psychiatry as a career. The effectiveness of the program was reported as the strategy to increase interest in psychiatry, encouraging students to pursue psychiatry as a career.

RANZCP Psychiatry Interest Forum was established in 2014, which has significant impact on, supporting recruitment into psychiatry. 5000 medical students and medical practitioners have joined it, since its inception, and 3000 are, active members in Australia and New Zealand. 859 members have transitioned into RANZCP training program who have either completed or progressing towards Fellowship (www.ranzcp. org/pif).

ANZJP and AP

RANZCP was further complemented by the birth of monthly **Australian New Zealand Journal of psychiatry (ANZJP)** in 1967 with its phenomenal contribution to Australian Psychiatry and its ever-increasing international impact. Bimonthly **Australasian Psychiatry journal** was established in 1993. Both these peer-reviewed journals have maintained widespread interest around the world with excellent global ranking.

ANZJP achieved impressive impact factor of 5.08, ranking it, as the leading psychiatric journal in the Asia Pacific region, and Southern Hemisphere, and 18th among psychiatric journals worldwide. The impact factor is calculated as the total number of citations to papers published in the ANZJP over the last 2 years divided by the total number of paper published during that time (Raj Gopal S 2017).

The current editors of both the journals Prof Malhi and Prof Brakoulias ought to be congratulated, for maintaining the global ranking and strength of clinical and academic culture of Australian psychiatry, through the journals.

Australia's international psychiatrists

There is no dearth of impressive academic environment to train outstanding psychiatric workforce in Australia.

Prof Gordon Parker published an impressive account of **Australian psychiatrists** *on world stage* (Parker G 2020) including stalwarts like John Cade, Aubrey Lewis, Leslie Kiloh, B Carroll and Issy Pilowsky. John Cade was the most influential Australian psychiatrist, for taking the first step towards ending the asylum system, by his advent of psychopharmacology: the rediscovery of lithium, which still remains the gold standard and has changed the medical treatment for mentally ill for ever. These were the names, which set the place of Australian psychiatry, on the world map and became the role model and inspiration, for the future generations of psychiatrists, who excel both nationally and internationally to keep the 'Dream Alive'.

I was extremely fortunate to have worked with Prof Leslie Kiloh as his registrar at Callan Park Neuropsychiatric Institute (NPI), a state-wide, specialist mental health service in NSW, of which he was the director. I later worked as his registrar and senior registrar at the newly opened psychiatric unit of Prince of Wales Hospital in late 70s. It was difficult to accept him as a colleague and not a mentor when we both worked as part-time members of Mental Health Review Tribunal many years later. A softly spoken, courteous: a true gentleman fitted my ideal image of a Guru whose, every word of imparted knowledge, sealed in my professional foundation. Despite his humility, thoughtfulness and generosity his leadership was never in doubt.

His review, titled "Pseudo–dementia" was a classic: published in Acta Psychiatrica Scandinavica, and remained as one of the most cited papers for many years (Kiloh LG 1961). The paper was practical and lucid and was widely acclaimed.

Pseudo–dementia was not the term he coined but revived for the benefit of my generation.

His 1961 book on electro-encaphalography was another classic.

In the same year he published one of the earliest outcome studies of then recently introduced imipramine. For many years he co-authored with Sir Martin Roth: The British Encyclopaedia of Medical Practice. The other eponymous as a neurologist to his credit was Kiloh-Nevin Syndrome: anterior interosseous nerve syndrome (one of the median nerve entrapment).

A neurologist turned psychiatrist, Prof Kiloh emigrated from UK in 1962 to take up the position of the first professor of psychiatry at the University of New South Wales.

Leslie Kiloh's influence on academic Australian psychiatry cannot be overestimated (Parker G. 1997).

It was a fitting tribute to name the new 50 bed psychiatric unit at Sydney's Prince of Wales Hospital as the Kiloh Centre in 2000.

Another significant name, in the list, was Eric Cunnigham Dax, a British born Australian psychiatrist, who was head of the Victorian Mental Health Authority, though he may not be truly an academic. His greatest legacy was his dedication to art therapy. Cunningham Dax collection is the tribute to his work, which is, one of the largest, collection in the world along with Musee Art Brute in Lausanne, Switzerland and Prinzhorn collection in Heidelberg Germany. It houses, over 16,000, art-work created by people with an experience of mental illness and trauma. The art includes work on paper, paintings and photographs, poems, textile, journals and digital media. A commendable initiative, is not only to raise awareness and reduce stigma towards mental illnesses through art, but it also uncover the talents of a person for his /her renewed self worth.

The excellence of academic work remains unfulfilled till it is translated into patient care. Unfortunately we lag behind, in providing the desired services to our patients, which may be a complex issue despite our highly trained and dedicated professionals and technology. The decline of public mental health services has an impact on the psychiatric services, which depends on psychiatrists and trainees, for delivering formal and informal clinical teaching, as well as research, besides their clinical role. With recent adverse publicity of declining resources of public health system, in addition to slow progress in preparing early career academics, will be a challenge, in maintaining the high standards of academic psychiatry, we have taken for granted.

Already there are concerns for academic psychiatrist; becoming an endangered species with its potential impact on undergraduate teaching, postgraduate training, research capacity and academic advice on health policies (Henderson S, et al. 2014).

With the globalisation of education and required financial needs, there is international awareness to attract students, making academic institutions more commercial, engaged in media, marketing and promotions. Nevertheless mentoring as a core of academic responsibility, in appropriate scientific environment, must be fiercely defended.

The most important and challenging role RANZCP has: to prepare the future generations of competent and sensitive psychiatrists, to meet the needs of the contemporary society. It has continued to reform the teaching and learning; in keeping with research and experience: much different to my training in early 70s based on traditional learning methods. The passive information transfer via, lectures have come under considerable criticism in the recent decades, particularly for the development of higher order thinking and skills. Retention of information is problematic in lectures with students' attention span consistently found at 70% in the first 10 minutes and 20% in the final 20 minutes. Several large systematic reviews and meta-analyses support the effectiveness of active learning techniques in science and higher education (Kumar S, et al 2017).

Flipped classroom: a relatively new concept, with the advent of information technology. The learning material is prepared, before the face-to-face active learning, which appears to be more effective.

In late 2012 RANZCP introduced Competency Based Fellowship Program (CBFP) and Work Based Activities to produce the next generation of psychiatrists. This apprenticeship model facilitates the interaction between the supervisors and the trainees, addressing organisational as well as clinical skills. Trainees need to develop communications skills, critical appraisal and reflective skills.

The examination consists of Extended Multiple Choice Questions, Modified Essay Questions and Observed Structured Clinical Examination.

Psychotherapy must remain the core skill of a psychiatrist. With this in mind the College utilised the Australian Government's Specialist Training Position initiative, in creating a psychotherapy registrar position. The dedicated trainee position, provides the opportunities for honing the psychotherapeutic skills with patient, supervision and professional development aligned together.

Academic mission of research, teaching and clinical excellence has underpinned the quality of health care for over 100 years (Pennington DG 2008).

CPD

In order to improve and maintain the quality of clinical and academic standards, College introduced mandatory Continuing Professional Development (CPD) program in 1996. The significant part of **CPD** is Peer Review Group. It is a small self–selected group of peers, who meet to review their work, in a setting that is organised to be supportive, for the individuals involved, to present and learn from the presentations of their work experiences and issues. The merit of the program was realised in its adoption by other Colleges both from within and outside Australia.

The effective practice of modern psychiatry is becoming increasingly dependent on the outputs of health and medical research. Research and quality improvements are important in the process of improving clinical practice.

Conducting clinical mentoring project is the key role of academic psychiatry, which has become increasingly challenging in the changing environment of higher education and health system. Therefore it needs to be acknowledged, as part of clinical duties throughout their careers, in terms of funding, designated availability of time, as well as a senior and experienced clinical researcher to groom the new generation of researchers. I often felt that I missed out on the opportunity of a mentor who could have guided me in the direction, I once cherished.

Research activities should be built in, as part of undergraduate and Fellowship training programs. It should be made into an attractive career path, not restricted to academic centers at major universities. The remarkable pace of neuroscience growth demands active engagement of our future psychiatrists with the broad discipline of neuroscience and genetics.

Scholarly Project was introduced in 2012, as part of the training program to provide opportunities for the prospective researchers, fostering crucial clinical curiosity. It involves a trainee undertaking an original research, in an area, relevant to psychiatry. Scholarship is one of the core competencies expected of all trainees on completion of RANZCP Fellowship program. As a scholar, the trainee needs to demonstrate a lifelong commitment to reflective learning, as well as the creation, dissemination, application and translation of medical knowledge (Royal College Framework).

Mentoring supervision of a research project can be, immensely rewarding, for clinical psychiatrist supervisors and their supervisees.

In medicine, research can't stand alone without clinical collaboration therefore most of the academic positions are offered with dual responsibilities. To accomplish the role of a researcher, the person needs to be highly motivated and focused as the research demands time, energy and commitment, beyond the call of duty.

Evidence Based Medicine

Evidence based medicine: paradigm for modern professional practice of psychiatry is now, the global gold mark of translating any research into clinical activity. Evidence based care would cost no more than treatment as usual, but will increase health gains by two-thirds (Andrews G, et al. 2003).

Randomised controlled trials (RCTs), meta-analysis and systematic reviews are important contributions, to clinical practice as well as contributing to evidence based medicine. Controlled randomised trials are, regarded as the gold standard, well above the observational studies or clinical anecdotes, although it cannot control the unknown variables. However the interpretation of RCTs, in some studies have been found to have, opposing conclusions.

Meta-analysis have also, been flawed for being inconsistent.

Lower ranking in the hierarchy of evidence, observational Studies are contaminated by confounding variables and circumstances across time.

Anecdotes though educationally illustrative are subject to bias.

Most of us have learnt not to accept, all the scientific information blindly, without subjecting it to the critical appraisal of our common sense (Little J D, et al. 2019).

So there can be many unforeseeable variables, which can impact on the outcome, making it approximate, rather than absolute

Another interesting example was that we were taught as undergraduates the theory of peptic ulcer as 'hurry worry and curry' to the exclusion of any external organism. It all changed with the chance discovery of evidence based Helicobacter Pylori in gastric ulcers revolutionising the treatment (Marshall BJ. 2002).

The quest for clinically translatable biomarkers in psychiatry, have come on the forefront of research activities. Australia is making headways in this direction, despite the paucity of researchers. Brain imaging has yet to achieve clinical diagnostic or prognostic use. Pharmacogenetics is another field waiting for the momentum. Matching genetic profile of the patient with pharmacological profile of the medication will be a huge step in patient outcome. Pharmaco-genetics, unfortunately has not yet established as a valid clinical tool in psychiatry.

There have been repeated concerns expressed both in Australia and around the world that there is systematic bias to the publication of positive findings and failure to publish negative results. The obvious reasons are; the support of pharmaceutical industry and, for the journal and the author: more citations. To address the problem; in 2005, the International Committee of Medical Journal Editors mandated that clinical-trials, should be, prospectively registered as a condition of publication (Porter RJ, et al. 2017).

References

Andrews G, Sanderson K, et al. 2003. Cost effectiveness of current and optimal treatment for schizophrenia. British Journal of Psychiatry 183: 427-435.

Henderson S, Porter RJ, et al. 2014. Why academic psychiatry is endangered. ANZJP 49:9-12.

Kiloh LG. Pseudo-dementia. Acta Psychiatrica Scandinavica 1961;37: 336-351.

Kumar S, McLean L, et al. Incorporating active learning in psychiatry education. Australasian Psychiatry 2017 Vol 25 (3) 304-309.

Little J D, Davidson L, et al. Clinically, what ought we to believe? Australasian Psychiatry 2019 Vol 27(1) 72-74.

Marshall BJ. The discovery, that Helicobacter pylori, a spiral bacterium caused peptic ulcer disease. Helicobacter pioneers. Melbourne: Blackwell Science Asia 2002: 165202.

Parker G Australian psychiatrists *on world stage* (ANZJP 2020, Vol. 54(1) 15-19.

Parker G. Obituary. Leslie Gordon Kiloh. Australasian Psychiatry 1997; 5: 250-251.

Pennington DG 2008. Physician-leaders and hospital performance: Is there an association? Social Science and Medicine 73: 535-539.

Porter RJ, Boden JM, et al. Failure to publish negative results: A systematic bias in psychiatric literature. ANZJP 2017 Vol 51 (3) 212-214.

Raj Gopal S 2017 Impact factors and psychiatric journals: An international perspective. BJ Psych International14: 15-18.

Robertson T, Walter G, et al. Medical students' attitude towards a career in psychiatry before and after viewing a promotional DVD. Australasian Psychiatry 2009; 17: 311-317.

Royal College Framework. Available at htpp://www.royalcollege.ca/ portal/page/portal/ rc/canmeds/ framework.

MEDICAL BOARD

DOCTORS ARE ONE of the, most esteemed group, of people in the community and most of the doctors naturally earn that honour, by their dedication, commitment, service and conscience. People form the most trusting relationship with their doctors, putting their life in the hands of the doctors, which is suitably acknowledged and reciprocated by most of us. Most doctors do not take our role lightly and view it, as one of the greatest privileges of life, responding to it with utmost sincerity. As medical professionals we are trained to suppress our distress, to preserve our functioning, but this defence may break down under cumulative stressors, fatigue and lack of organisational support. Altruism: caring for their patients without concern about reward, still ranks highly for their motivation.

Medical profession by its nature has within it, the realm of inexhaustible agenda of self-improvement and life long learning. It is further reinforced by the cultural norm of professional environment. Nevertheless there can be bad apples, to smear the image. As human health remains the highest priority for each and every one, there is no room for complacency when dealing with someone else's health. To ensure that all the doctors remain on the path of near perfection of their role, a regulating body is essential to oversee and objectively evaluate the services we provide and the outcome.

Unfortunately the national medical board and state councils have taken their role of protecting the patient, with tunnel vision and predetermined notion that unless absolutely proven otherwise, the doctor is at fault. Therefore the course of their enquiry from the outset is predetermined for the validation of issues, presented by the patient, and against the doctor.

Demand for increasing unconditional accountability by the registration authority that solely relies on, patient's complaints, rather than reality, practicality, or circumstances, to protect the patient, has changed the culture of compassionate and meaningful autonomy in the best interest of the patient. It has generated a new class of defensive medicine where from the outset the doctor must be mindful of possible legal repercussions of his/her actions and decisions. Some of these may be fair and necessary but some may not.

Doctors' surveys around the country have repeatedly revealed that their worst fear is to be contacted by the medical board. Most agreed with board's dictatorial and uncompromising position.

As past president of Australian Indian Medical Graduate Association and, in my role as a practicing psychiatrist, I became familiar with many doctors who were either rightly or wrongly reprimanded by the Medical Council. The two cases I illustrate here left me with sadness, unable to comprehend the fairness of regulating body.

Dr X

Dr X was referred to see me with a fortnight of severe depression where he was ruminating on suicide. His wife did not feel confident to care for him at home. So I decided to hospitalise him. His wife arranged for a locum when he stopped going to work a week earlier. He isolated himself and spoke very little. As the story unfolded, he was, taken aback by a letter, from the Medical Council, that a couple of his female patients have accused him of sexual misconduct. A spiritual man, devoted husband and father of 3 young children, the nature of allegation was furthest from his mind. With no recollection of any contact, remotely sexual, he responded to the letter. Unfortunately his response was disregarded and more investigations commenced to validate the complaint against him. The case went on for several years. My reports were amongst many others with objective and fair appraisal. During the course of legal proceedings he was granted conditional privilege to see the patients with a female chaperon, which was, later withdrawn. He was given weekend prison sentence with its profound impact on his young children. The complainants withdrew their initial complaint, changing it to their dissatisfaction with his service, without elaborating on it. The Council maintained that he lacked the feelings of remorse and guilt, (for the alleged crime he maintained, he never committed) a psychopathic trait: most unsuitable in his role as a doctor, and as the result of it he was deregistered. Life changed. His young children became adults. Two of them studied law to understand his plight and possible defense of their father. Dr X, a proud man from a well educated family and excellent academic record himself, succumbed to disability pension for his chronic depression falling from his grace. Disillusioned with the law of the land, all his children along with their mother moved to US. Both his daughters suffered from recurring depression. His wife suffered from Cancer and died. He himself moved to US though needed to return to Australia to maintain his Australian pension, his only source of income. Living with his children was not easy, so he divided his time between his birth country, Australia his adopted country and US the country of his final journey.

Dr Z

The 2nd case, which moved me, was; of a well reputed, conscientious, competent and committed doctor. I saw her on strictly confidential terms.

A patient's disgruntled daughter who was doctor Z's ex patient lodged a complaint that her 52 years old mother Mrs M was poorly cared for, by the doctor with wrong diagnosis and wrong treatment.

Mrs M was referred to doctor Z a few years ago, with a diagnosis of attention-deficit disorder by another doctor, upon his retirement. Mrs M was treated with dexamphetamine for many years. As doctor Z could not justify the diagnosis, the stimulant was gradually withdrawn despite resistance from the patient. Mrs M had a long standing history of substance abuse and multiple hospitalisations dating back to her adolescence. She met her husband in the drug circle and they continued with their drug habits. At some stage doctor Z also saw one of Mrs M's son when he was charged for possession of illegal drugs. Both her marriage and family life were riddled with problems. Mrs M accused her husband of sexually molesting their 2 youngest children when doctor Z involved child protection unit of the Department of Community Services. For his revenge her husband called the local community health services about her alleged delusional thinking and being fearful for himself and, the children. With the arrival of the police and ambulance she was petrified, and resisted being handcuffed. The more she resisted, becoming more aggressive, the more it validated her husband's claim of her apparent psychotic presentation. She was restrained and physically pushed against her will, in to the back of the police van, which she found extremely humiliating, and it became her recurring nightmare. She was diagnosed by the hospital as suffering from schizophrenia: based on the symptoms her husband narrated, and her aggressive and abusive outburst, retaliating against her forced admission. This appeared the beginning of the end for this lady. The family used her involuntary hospitalisation as a punitive measure whenever they thought she needed it, at their discretion and they quickly learnt the process to make it happen. As it is customary, most of the public patients are reviewed by rotating trainees, and the diagnosis is generally based on previous diagnosis, as well as the collateral information discounting the patient who is considered out of mind. Independent evaluation by experienced doctor may not be always possible. Unfortunately for the patient, a life long trajectory: life of psychosis begins.

Mrs M was given almost continuous Community Treatment Orders requiring, long acting antipsychotic medications. She suffered from severe side effects, which were sidelined, with no attention given to it. She lost faith in public health system and did not wish to see anyone unless forced by legal orders. With some difficulty and hope of being reviewed independently, she agreed to see doctor Z. They gradually developed a trusting therapeutic relationship and agreed not to be persuaded by the family, but to make objective and independent assessment, should she ever require care against her will or involuntary hospitalisation of least restrictive manner. Mrs M was a responsible woman who took good care of her 2 young children, far younger than her 3 older ones. She only displayed 'delusional' thinking in response to the marital or family conflicts. Due to her fear and trauma related to her forced hospitalisations, doctor Z avoided hospitalisation as much as possible, and considered the diagnosis of borderline personality disorder, though continued with low dosage oral anti psychotic medication which appeared to stabilise her.

Returning back to the complaint. Medical Council rejected the comprehensive response from doctor Z and decided to take further action by subjecting doctor Z to an interview. The 2 interviewers from Medical Council confirmed the allegations, stating that the doctor was impaired, rather than give a fair appraisal of the management process, doctor Z followed. Their report condemned the doctor as incompetent and too dangerous to remain in practice. The diagnosis given by the interviewing panel, with their superficial knowledge of the patient history was, Erotomania based on Mrs M's interest in her newly arrived neighbour who was recently divorced. Doctor Z feeling surprised, by this diagnosis, could have disputed it, but it was not her place to do so. This was followed by another assessment at Dr Z's office by a visiting team of 4 members who randomly selected patients' files to examine, and joined in the live patients' consultations. This was again to confirm that doctor Z bitterly failed on all the parameters required for registration. No evidence was taken from the multidisciplinary team involved, or the patient herself, who was lucid and logical, capable of providing her own evidence. Doctor Z was given the option to complete a clinical retraining program and undergo neuropsychological assessment or surrender medical registration to avoid being deregistered, an unthinkable option for any doctor. Dr Z, a vibrant personality was a multi skilled, multitalented person who was actively and passionately involved in clinical and academic activities including, published books and papers in medical and nonmedical fields and providing highly appreciated service to her patients for several decades. A proud person, doctor Z could not share the story of falling from the grace, with anyone but myself. Doctor Z knew that I was unable to help her, but I was hoping that sharing with me perhaps, will give her, the courage to start a new chapter, on the ashes of her lost professional life. I was hoping that her true happiness, in winning this most challenging time of her life, will come from her good inner life, from disposition of mind and soul and being honest and truthful to her patients.

It takes reflection, contemplation and self-discipline to accept damage.

On our last meeting neither of us felt any need to speak. We hugged with teary eyes and parted.

The pandemic crisis of Covid-19 has given weight, not to take even an invisible enemy for granted. Doctor Z's journey of downfall began, with an unassuming simple young woman, who dictated the course of the professional decision, ending an illustrious career and a productive life. Mrs M was angry and remorseful on learning of the complaint her daughter lodged, against her trusted doctor when Dr Z declined to see her.

Mrs M was hopeful of rebuilding her life with help from Dr Z, in whom she finally found a trustworthy not only a therapist, but a mentor as well.

Medical culture remains deeply rooted both by custom and training, in high standards of autonomous individual performance (Leape L 2055).

Blame may offer expiation of unconscious guilt: a simplified evaluation of complex situation. Clinicians are the likely target of the patient's or their family's unrealistic expectations. Some personality styles are prone to uncritical blaming behaviours, seeking retribution in the form of dismissal, humiliation or persecution of those, they blame for adverse events (Lester G, et al. 2004).

There is growing literature, on the effects on clinicians, involved in the adverse events of litigation and, from the work done on the effects of, shame and guilt on the immune system (Nash L, et al. 2007).

It is not just, to hold a prudent clinician culpable, if they are trying their best to use their skills, care and knowledge to provide a service. Disciplinary decision making-strategies may be outcome based, rule based and risk based. Culpable clinician actions must be firm, if possible reparative, but not overtly punitive or humiliating.

There is little relationship between successful litigation, and the extent, to which the negligence contributed, to the harm suffered.

A fair and transparent health culture must equally include patients and the doctors. There should be better management of unreasonable and querulously litigious complainants, which consumes countless human and financial health resources.

References

Leape L and Birwick. Five years after to err is human: What have we learnt? JAMA 2005; 293: 2384-2390.

Lester G, Wilson B, et al. Unusually persistent complainants. British Journal of Psychiatry 2004 184: 352-356.

Nash L, Daly M et al. Psychological morbidity in Australian doctors who have and have not experienced a medico-legal matter. ANZJP 2007; 41: 917-925.

MENTAL HEALTH OF INDIGENOUS AUSTRALIANS

ACCORDING TO 2016 Australian census, an estimated 798,365 Aboriginal and Torres Strait Islander people were in Australia, representing 3.3 percent of total Australian population. It was reduced to 745.000 in 2020 or 3.0 percent of the total population. Indigenous Australians have significantly greater challenges and disadvantages as compared to non-Indigenous people in the areas of socioeconomic factors, life expectancy, health and high level of psychological distress. They have significantly raised incidence of chronic illnesses including respiratory, metabolic and cardiac pathology. Their life expectancy is over ten years less than non-Indigenous population.

There are 3 times more suicides, reported among Indigenous people, against the national data. Psychotic disorders are common and more so among young adult Aboriginal men, with high rates of comorbid conditions including substance use, intellectual impairment and diabetes (Hunter E, et al. 2011). A population based study of Indigenous children and adolescents in Western Australia found that 24 percent Indigenous children were at the high risk of clinically significant emotional and behavioural difficulties and further 11.4 percent at moderate risk. In the age range of 12-17 years 20.5 percent were at high risk against 7 percent of non-Indigenous adolescents (Blair et al. 2005). In this study 9 percent females and 4.1 percent males reported attempted suicide.

Communities along Australia's northern coastline, home of some of the world's most intact Aboriginal cultures, are caught in the epidemic of child suicide and self harm that has claimed at least 50 young lives in the last decade. The suicide rate among, under 25 years, was almost 4 times the national average. The youngest recorded victim was a 10 years old boy. There has been a strong feeling that outside constructs imposed on the traditional societies had left people feeling powerless and unable to cope.

Depression, anxiety, and drug and alcohol abuse are the most common, diagnoses. Alcohol and substance abuse are twice as prevalent among, Indigenous population as it is in non-Indigenous population. Australian government endeavours to provide culturally appropriate health services. Despite concerted national effort to enhance mainstream primary care service and substantial gains in accessing mental health care for Indigenous people, it has remained a critical issue in Australia (Jorm AF, et al 2013).

Both Australia and Canada shared the dilemma of caring for their Indigenous population. The Stolen Generation were, the children of Australian Aboriginal and Torres Strait Islander descent, who were removed from their families by the Australian federal and state government agencies and church missions, under act of their respective parliaments. The goals of the scheme were dictated by the rules of the country that considered Aboriginal community and parenting: savage and unsuitable for modern society. The children were separated from their families to socialize them to the values, beliefs and habits of the colonial society and merge them with non-Aboriginal world. Both countries paid heavily for their culturally insensitive dictatorial actions, though not more than the victims of trans-generational cycle of neglect, abuse, violence, dysfunction and mental illness.

Colonisation of Aboriginal land, by British invaders, had the most devastating effect, on the traditional culture and family values of Indigenous people, who lived in harmony for thousands of years, and have never come to terms with the disintegration of their kinship system, and family units, which has changed forever.

Lack of acknowledgement of people's existence, in country's constitution, had major impact on their sense of identity and value within the community: perpetuating discrimination and prejudice, further eroding the hope of Indigenous people. This is associated with socio-economic disadvantage, and higher rates of, mental and physical illnesses and incarcerations.

Australian constitution was written in 1890s against a backdrop of racism, which led to White Australia policy and a range of other discriminatory laws and practices. Many of these practices and laws were not specifically directed against Indigenous people but other Chinese and non-white immigrants to Australia like myself. Embedded in Australian legal system was the capacity, for racial discrimination, determining everything from their intelligence to suitability for certain roles.

Australian Constitution

In 1901, casting them as dying race, Australian constitution excluded Aboriginal natives when counting the number of people living in the country. Sir Edmund Burton the first prime minister of Australia, in Constitutional Convention of 1898: made it clear that federal government needed the power to regulate the affairs of the people of 'coloured or inferior races like Chinaman, Japanese, Hindus and other barbarians who are in the Commonwealth'. The strong government policy maintained the race-based distinction.

Recognising Indigenous people in the constitution has been the subject, of lengthy analysis and debate. After well over a century, the last element of racial discrimination is yet to be removed from the most important Australian law: The Constitution (Williams G.2015).

RANZCP has played a significant role with the reintegration, of the Aboriginal and Torres Islander people back, into the main-stream culture. In addition to its Reconciliation Action Plan, it has also become the partner of Recognise: a people's movement, to recognise Aboriginal and Torres Islander peoples, in Australian Constitution, and to remove racially discriminatory provisions from it.

References

Blair EM, Zubrick SR, et al. (2005) The Western Australian Aboriginal Child Health Survey: findings to date on adolescents. MJA 183; 433-435.

Hunter E, Gynther B, et al. Psychosis and its correlates in a remote Indigenous population RANZJP 2011 Vol 9 No 5.

Jorm AF, Malhi G S Evidence based mental health services reform in Australia: Where to next? ANZJP 2013. 47: 693-695.

Williams G. Why its time to recognise Indigenous people in the Constitution. ANZJP 2015, Vol 23 (3) 214-217.

HUMAN RIGHTS OF MENTALLY ILL PEOPLE

HUMAN RIGHTS VIOLATION has been a long-standing issue around the world in relation to mentally ill people, which has led to many enquiries and Royal commissions. The current trend internationally is for empowering the consumer to play major role in their approach to mental health treatment. Consistent with this, the Human Rights Act was reformed in 2013 to include decision-making capacity. The requirement since then has been for the clinician to monitor the decision-making capacity of the patient, before applying for his/her involuntary status. This is in line with United Nations Convention on the Rights of the Persons with Disability. Unfortunately it has not been fully implemented. In 2015 the legislation that regulates involuntary treatment in NSW, was amended, to provide, that clinicians should make every effort, which is reasonably practicable, to obtain the consent of people with mental illness or mental disorder, when developing treatment plan and recovery plan for their care (Mental Health Act 2007 NSW). By involving the patient, as a partner in making the treatment plan, the doctor emphasises and reinforces the patient's strength, as a person, instead of their weakness in a dependent sick role, thus opening up the doors to more flexible, appropriate responsible and responsive outcome.

The provision of advance directive, specifies person's treatment preferences should they lose their decision making capacity in the future. It allows flexibility within acceptable clinical reasoning to manage the emergent-clinical situation during an episode of mental illness. It empowers the patient who can ask the reason for deviating from the advance directives.

The concept that mentally ill people have the same human rights as everyone else: is more accepted today than a few decades ago. Psychiatrists have to be on the forefront, dispelling myths and breaking down the barriers of stigma and discrimination by strong advocacy for human rights.

Shared decision-making is yet another step towards autonomy of the patient. It has potential benefit in improving medication attitude and adherence with treatment. Enhanced autonomy from shared decision making may also make the patient feel valued and empowered.

Australian Government Productivity Commission Mental Health enquiry 2020, has advocated people centered system, emphasizing that people should have real choices, in managing their own mental health, and be empowered to choose the treatment and supports, that are right for them, across full spectrum of clinical and non-clinical needs.

Euthanasia

Euthanasia though as old as the human history: has only been formally recognised in the last few decades, for open discussion. It has been unethical for the most part of the history of medicine. The first jurisdiction in the world to legalise euthanasia was, in Northern Territory of Australia. Since then most countries have adopted the legalisation of physician assisted suicide including Australian state of Victoria in recognition of quality of life against its painful prolongation. The current criteria for euthanasia, includes grievous and irremediable medical condition. Overall the debate in general, continues in Australia, without making a, legislation at national level.

Official Visitors

Official Visitors are people experienced in mental health treatment and care. They are appointed by NSW Minister of Heath to visit people in the mental health inpatient facility and are able to assist with community treatment orders. It aims to safeguard the standards of treatment, care, rights and dignity of people being treated under the NSW Mental Health Act 2007 while maintaining an independent community perspective. The Official visitors are also accessible to family, friends, staff and other people interested in the care of the patient. At least quarterly audit by the official visitor, of all documents related to the patient, ensures its timely and comprehensive completion.

Mental Health Commission

Long standing demand in the community, for mental health reform led to the birth of Mental Health Commission in 2011, following extensive consultation process. Its objective was to create independent body, that would take a holistic approach, addressing the needs of the people, with mental illness, across the government and whole of life, and deal with related diseases and disorders as a big picture.

Mental Health Review Tribunal (MHRT)

Involuntary treatment of people with mental illness is, one of the most controversial practices in medicine, which was traditionally provided within the long-stay psychiatric hospitals. The shift to community based psychiatric services, for all ages, has been essential in de-stigmatising and modernising the treatment of mentally ill. With increasing emphasis on human rights specially, for people with mental illness, it was adopted to deliver the appropriate services in the least restrictive environment, which led to community based, mental health and Community Treatment Orders.

Although it had been operational in almost invisible form for many years, it was not until 1990 when it expanded into its current active role under the Mental Health Act 2007 and Mental Health (Forensic Provisions) Act 1990. I worked as a part time member for over 25 years involved in the following functions of the Tribunal.

Reviewing cases of detained persons to determine if they should continue to be detained in the hospital.

Hearing appeals against refusal of, a medical superintendent to discharge a patient

Making orders for financial management where people are unable to make competent decisions for themselves due to a mental illness.

Determining applications for treatments and surgery on detained patients.

Making, revoking or varying community counseling and community treatment orders.

Determining person's fitness for further trial after the jury has found the person unfit.

The release or disposition of a person, acquitted of crime, by reason of mental illness.

Making Community Treatment Orders for the involuntary patients, following their discharge from the hospital, for providing least restrictive community based treatment, for a specified time frame.

Introduction of 21st century technology made the Hearings of MHRT more efficient and cost effective with wider coverage of the entire state.

By world standard, Community Treatment orders in Australia, are much higher and are rising though with considerable variation across states (Light EM 2019). It is inconsistent with Australian ratification of United Nations Convention on The Rights of person with Disability including those with mental illness, declared in 2014.

United Nations has highlighted the involuntary treatment in Australia commenting that Australia should repeal all legislation that authorises imposition of compulsory treatment either in the hospital or in the community.

A Cochrane review of international randomised controlled trials showed no evidence that CTOs improved social functioning, mental state or quality of life, hospital readmission rates or reduction in health services use (Kinsey SR et al).

Any change takes a long time to infuse in mental health system, like Australian jurisdiction introducing reforms, of patient's decision making capacity test, to deny an offered treatment as patients' right, and to minimise compulsory treatment. Human interaction is the fundamental basis upon which psychiatry is built. Empowering autonomy is an important step towards equal recognition, before the law.

Seclusion of involuntary patients has been a contentious issue for a long time. Reducing and where possible eliminating the use of seclusion/restrain is a policy priority, for reforms in Australian mental health care. There is a need for broader analysis of all coercive or restrictive practices, to ensure that reductions in seclusion events are not achieved by substitution with other restrictive practices like mechanical, chemical or physical restrain.

It is even more important in a child and adolescent inpatient area: traumatic for both staff and the patient. Most of the patients feel humiliated, frightened confused depressed, angry and punished. As an alternative, collaborative problem solving behavioural management can help to uncover the root cause of the behaviour. It is useful to identify the underlying deficits in executive functioning, emotional regulation, communication, social skills and cognitive flexibility.

The issue of competent people being forced to accept treatment, as does the issue, of those not competent to consent, being treated without any, additional protection of their rights, remains on the agenda. Greater autonomy to people with mental illness must be considered as part of their comprehensive recovery.

Involuntary treatments like CTO should be restricted to only those patients who lack decision making capacity and yet need protection for their own safety

Guardianship Legislation

When a person with impaired decision making capacity has no carer or substitute decision maker, needs medical or psychiatric care in a hospital and refuses treatment, a public guardian is appointed. Australian states and territories have guardianship legislation that provides measures to make decisions about people who have decision-making disability.

NGO

The National Mental Health Plan recognised the increasing delivery of community based mental health services via **Non-Government Organisations (NGO)** allocating them substantial funding to assist people with severe mental illnesses. Some of their major projects have been rehabilitation program like independent living skills, healthy living, fitness, stress management, social skills and creative activities. Unfortunately only about 25% people utilised these services.

Pioneer Clubhouse is a, community based service run by an NGO. There are more than 300 Clubhouses worldwide 10 of which are in Australia. Clubhouse adheres to a common approach known as the Clubhouse model, which includes helping a person with mental illness to return to their optimal level of functioning. Pioneer Clubhouse members also use government and private services, for clinical and medical aspects of their psychiatric care (Macleod V. 2005).

The Schizophrenia Fellowship is another well-known NGO, of NSW Inc. It provides psychosocial rehabilitation program for people recovering from mental illness.

Unfortunately there is no reliable measure of NGO services, as the outcome measured, do not reflect the program goals. Even with all the funding, education and focus, data are not being routinely collected, and are unlikely to be usable to show effectiveness of services and programs (Kightley M, et al. 2010).

I was involved in **Compeer program** with good results. It is a non-profit, volunteer-friendship program for people living with mental illness. It complements the treatment of people with severe mental illness through social integration, employing both educational and interpersonal contact, to combat the burden of stigma. It is the quality rather than length of the Compeer friendship that makes a difference to attitudes.

Mental Health Carers Australia was formerly known as ARAFMI (Association of Relatives and Friends of Mentally Ill) It is the national advocacy group concerned with the wellbeing, and promotion of the needs of the families and carers, supporting someone with mental illness. It provides national voice for families and carers, to enable the best possible life by influencing systemic changes in government policies and service provider practice, to improve the family and carer experience of the mental heath system

Mental Health co-responder program

At least 20% of all mental health referrals to the emergency department of any large hospital will come from police (Lee S, et al. 2008).

This is a relatively new program to resolve immediate mental health crises, minimising its escalation in the community. It involves co-responder: a mental health nurse, working alongside police, for on-site assessment. There is growing body of evidence both in Australia and overseas that timely access to mental health assessment and intervention provided through co-responder model averted ED presentation and hospital admissions (Lee S J, et al.2015).

Safety

World Health Organisation identifies patient safety as a serious global issue. In Australia 16.6 percent of all hospital inpatient episodes result in adverse events with at-least half of these being preventable. The same caution applies to the health professionals working for the patients specially, in the view of increasing hostility against doctors, and other health professionals in some countries.

Although the regular accreditation of hospitals does include safety measures, it should be further complemented with locally driven safety and quality improvement activities in consultation with frontline staff, patients, carers and health professionals.

References

Kightley M, Einfeld S, et al. Routine outcome measurement in mental health: feasibility for examining effectiveness of an NGO. Australasian Psychiatry April 2010 Vol 18 No 2. 167-169.

Kinsey SR et al Compulsory Community and Involuntary Outpatient Treatment for people with severe mental illness. Cochrane Database of Systemic Reviews 3: CD 004408.

Lee S, Brunero S, et al. Profiling police presentation of mental health consumers to an emergency department. Int J Ment Health Nurse 2008; 17: 311-316.

Lee S J, Thomas P et al. Outcome achieved by and police and clinician perspective on a joint police officer and mental health clinician mobile response unit. Int J Ment Health Nurs2015; 24: 538-546.

Light EM 2019 Rates of use of CTOs in Australia. International Journal of Law and Psychiatry 64:83-87.

Macleod V. Pioneer Spirit. The Story of Pioneer Clubhouse and its Partnership in Recovering from Mental Illness. Balgowla: Pioneer Clubhouse 2005.

FORENSIC PSYCHIATRY

DURING MY WORKING life, civil forensic psychiatry has not only become expansive, but complex, under the cover of medico-legal claims. It has also been compounded by, the deinstitutionalisation of 1970s. Significant minority of patients from the protection of, large institutions became exposed to adverse life circumstances, and antisocial life style. The relationship between aggression, and mental illness, became more apparent. The in-patient care of such patients is, either deliberately or inadvertently declined. With the growing number of mentally ill, and intellectually impaired offenders, the forensic resources are lagging behind. The proportion of Australians, in prison far exceeded the OECD average in 2018, at 167 per 100,000. Rapidly growing prison population combined with, high prevalence of psychiatric disorders amongst this group highlights the importance of ensuring, that there are adequate mental health service, to meet the need (Foulds JA. 2018).

More than one-third of Australian population born overseas, exceeding US, Canada and UK is reflected in the prison population with culturally and linguistically diverse background.

Medico-legal subdivision has been inundated with claims of Post Traumatic Stress Disorder both for its physical and psychological consequences. The symptoms of PTSD are generally subjective and the plaintiffs' perceptions are emotionally charged which may complicate the compensation issues. Undoubtedly it can lead to patient dissatisfaction and negative countertransference in the therapist.

With the expanding scope and practice of medico-legal work, many medico-legal companies have sprouted around the country, providing office space, secretarial support and referrals etc. So accredited report writing in these cases becomes a vital part of the practice of psychiatry. As this was not part of my training program, I learnt the art of high ethical standards, high level report writing skills, current knowledge of relevant legislation, good clinical knowledge and expressing my views within my expertise: by experience.

M'Naghten Rule

Defence on the grounds of insanity was formulated in 1843 as a reaction to the acquittal of, Daniel M'Naghten a Scottish wood turner, on the charges of murdering Edward Drummond an English civil servant (Prime minister's secretary) while suffering from paranoid delusions. He mistakenly shot Drummed instead of the UK Prime Minister Robert Peel. M'Naghten was a successful businessman and highly functional till the age of about 28 years. In 1841 he complained to various people that he was being persecuted by Tories and followed by their spies. He later told the court that he was compelled by the persecution destroying his peace of mind, which desperately drove him to the shooting. The court verdict was that M'Naghten was not a responsible or a reasonable person as his delusions of persecution deprived him of all restraint over his actions. He was not guilty on the ground of insanity.

'To establish a defence on the grounds of insanity, it must be clearly proved that, at the time of committing of the act, the party accused was labouring under such a defect of reason, from disease of mind, as not to know the nature and quality of the act he was doing, or if he did know it, that he did not know he was doing what was wrong"

The murder of colleagues

'Vengeance and retribution require a long time; it is the rule'
CHARLES DICKENS,
A tale of two cities

Dr T L

Crimes committed by psychiatric patients are not uncommon, but when it involves your brethren: it hits home.

On an unusually warm evening in late August I headed home after a busy day. Settled in the car for a long drive I started singing, an old favourite Hindi song, when I was, disturbed by the first news item, on the radio. A doctor in Blacktown (NSW) was stabbed to death by a patient. With no mobile phone I hurried to return home. My imagination was running wild thinking of doctors I knew in the area. Shaken as I was, rang my GP friend's home who worked in Blacktown. As I started to unload myself the phone rang. It was my secretary.

'Have you watched the news?' 'No'

'Quick put the TV on Dr T L was stabbed to death by his patient'

I did what I was asked to do, with a blank mind. I had no word to speak. My family watched every channel showing the story till late night. It distracted me from comprehending the full impact of the news. After a restless night I went to my clinic next morning, as I did not know what else I could do. He recently started working one day a week in my practice to relieve me, so that I could work as a research psychiatrist for NISAD: the schizophrenia research team at Prince of Wales hospital. He had a fully booked clinic on the day. The news of his murder was widespread. The patients turned up to share their shock and bewilderment, which I needed, as well, with people who respected my colleague. I then raced down in frenzy to the hospital 45 minutes away where we both worked, to talk and talk about the tragedy, sharing with the staff.

I met T at the beginning of my training in early 70s. We both were recent immigrants to the country soon after the end of white Australia policy, when overseas doctors were welcomed, to expand on the national health services. An easily noticeable charming man, both in his demeanour and personality, we found a lot in common to talk about, besides our training. As we worked in hospitals located on our way to the Institute of Psychiatry in Broughton Hall, we often shared our cars. After finishing the training T went to UK to get his MRC Psych, which was the usual practice for many psychiatrists at the time. We did not see each other for a few years till he returned to Sydney, and joined the hospital where I was a VMO. He later moved to live in the suburb where I was.

The night before the fateful day there was to be a grand round in the hospital, which often extended to late night. T's wife needed the car so she dropped him in the hospital and he was to travel home with me. We had a relaxing drive for more than an hour and had a lot, to talk on the topics of mutual interest. With the usual curtsies we parted after dropping him at his home. That was my last meeting with T.

Many years ago T saw this warring couple Mr and Mrs X. Mr X had unusual ideas, was uncompromising and socially isolative. He wanted, T to support him against his wife who was a well functioning reasonable person. These are the challenging situations, where remaining objective and honest, can be, misinterpreted as collusion, by a person of impaired mind. Mr X did not believe that T understood his plight and left. His wife consulted T a few more times till the couple parted. There was nothing unusual in this story for a psychiatrist, and no need for forced follow up.

After several years of separation Mr X gradually became preoccupied with his ex wife's whereabouts. This led to his belief that Dr T was instrumental in his marriage break up. He searched for Dr T for months and finally made an appointment to see him in Blacktown. On his way from Central Coast he started to become agitated and wanted to see someone as soon as possible. He drove to a hospital on his way. He needed to wait to see a psychiatrist and it was reported that he was, restless pacing the floor with some urgency. He left without seeing anyone and proceeded to his appointment in Blacktown. Dr T shared the rooms with other doctors and a pathology service. Mr X entered the consulting room at the appointed time. Soon after, a loud voice was heard outside the room. It seemed like an argument broke out where he accused Dr T for breaking his marriage, and wasn't prepared to listen to Dr T's clarification. He pulled a knife from his pocket stabbing the doctor who fled from his room into the kitchen through the waiting room followed by him. By the time the bewildered people around rushed to intervene, T was stabbed repeatedly, covered in blood with his last breath. Mr X went to his car changed his clothes and drove off.

With another senior colleague from the hospital, I attended the court most days of his trial hearings, for the cold-blooded execution Mr X committed. His defence of insanity was strong enough to commit him to a high security forensic institution. Years later as a member of mental health review tribunal I went to Morisset hospital for a scheduled hearing. Unbeknown to me Mr X was listed for a review. I needed to excuse myself for conflict of interest and was replaced by another psychiatrist on phone. I felt that my personal antagonism towards the man was likely to override my professional boundary.

Dr MT

In summing up his defence Dr J E G said 'Being murdered is: an occupational hazard as a psychiatrist'.

On 14th of October 2002, Dr MT a psychiatrist and a senior public servant was shot 4 times in an execution style shooting, in her Adelaide office building. Dr MT was well recognised for her determined reform of the psychiatric services in Australia. She equipped herself with formal qualification of MBA for effective managerial leadership and worked in positions of power in Victoria, NSW and finally in South Australia. After extensive and exhaustive investigations Dr J EG was charged 2 years later with Dr MT's murder.

Justice Ann Vanstone in handing down her judgement described the gravity of the crime as cool calculated and clever, which deserved extremely long non-parole period. Dr JEG was sentenced to 34 years of non-parole period dating back to 11 November 2002.

Both psychiatrists were outstanding in the pursuits of their success with exceptional academic background. They worked together at S G Hospital in Sydney, when Dr JEG started showing sign of disorganisation with tinge of paranoia, suspecting people of conspiring against him. Dr MT reported him to the medical board for harbouring possible psychiatric illness. This led to a series of assessments in the category of impaired registrants, which unfortunately exacerbated Dr JEG's suspicions and defiance, to safeguard his sanity. He was also riddled with somatic delusion of being HIV positive, despite many negative blood tests and consultations with 2 specialists. His self-diagnosed HIV was treated by his imported medications, at enormous cost.

Dr JEG was finally deregistered, killing his cherished dream of excelling as a professional and feeding into his determination to take revenge. Although the reason behind his deregistration was mental illness, his knowledge and performance in the trial, representing himself and cross examining the witnesses, as well as debating the law, surprised even the senior lawyers. He was in fine form and well controlled, with no doubt of his full mental functioning.

Psychiatry is more prone to uncertainties and differences of opinions than any other branch of medicine. Many people with mental illness are extremely bright and creative. It may also be the reason for the worse care; doctors with mental illness get, as they can disguise their problems avoiding enforced treatment. The dimensional nature of psychiatric diagnosis does not always make it easy to separate normal from abnormal thoughts. To some extent it is fed in our culture from very beginning of life like 'stranger danger' suspicion and the caution in trusting anyone specially, with the advent of technology, where virtual world often takes over the real world.

It is a matter of concern that whilst psychiatrists are in the business of de-stigmatising mental illness, when it comes to them personally they are secretive. Perhaps it is the matter for the College to ponder over it. In the case above we sadly lost 2 promising psychiatrists.

Schizophrenia was implicated in both of these murder charges. There is little doubt about the association between schizophrenia and homicide. To lesser extent is the evidence of bipolar affective disorder and violence. Danish birth cohort study and a case linkage study from Victoria found that women with affective psychosis were more in number and were often convicted for violent offences in comparison to their male counterparts. However this association was attributed to co-morbid substance abuse and environmental factors rather then the diagnosis of bipolar itself.

Massacre

Massacre is brutal and indiscriminate slaughter of many people. As safe as Australia seems to be, it has its own share of brutal killings of people unknown to the killer.

The Lindt Chocolate Café siege can come to any Australian mind as a relatively recent horror, which was a terrorist attack by a man named Man Haron Monis. A lone gunman held hostages, 10 customers and 8 employees of the Café, located in the center of Sydney city between 15th and 16th of December 2014 for 16 hours. 3 people died including Monis and 4 were physically injured. He was an Islamic extremist, had long standing history of antisocial personality and possibly a mental illness. He had strings of serious crime charges for violence both in his country of birth, and Australia.

Strathfield (a prestigious suburb of Sydney) **Plaza** on August 17, 1991 was the scene of, one of the most gruesome massacres in the history of NSW. The gunman Wade Frankum, a 33 years old taxi-driver, killed 8, including himself and injured 7 people, within 10 minutes, leaving 50 bullet casings littering the path of his shooting spree.

The coroner and the forensic psychiatrist believed that Frankum's action was impossible to predict as he had no criminal record and showed no sign of violence. He went to one of the high-ranking private schools. Nevertheless he was a sexual deviant who loved violence as revealed from the police search of his apartment, and from the statement of a prostitute he regularly visited. Although he was never formally diagnosed with a mental illness, he was a loner and an angry man with no friend. He expressed his anger to his sister and her boyfriend with whom he was sharing their deceased parents' apartment. His mother committed suicide 16 months earlier and he started to see a psychologist for depression for a couple of months early in 1991. He acquired shooter's licence, assault rifle, bowie knife and set of handcuffs between Jan and April 1991.

For me, the most important, irresponsible and appalling issue was the liberty of a common man to own any number of firearms without any restriction.

Thankfully the gun laws have changed, since then. In retrospect even if his sister raised alarm it may not have been easy to pin him down for treatment but may have been possible too.

Port Arthur Massacre: was country's worst mass murder on April 28-29th 1996 killing 35 people and wounding 18.

The gunman 28 years old Martin Bryant was later sentenced to 35 life terms. He was intellectually compromised and was on disability pension till by some fluke, he inherited large sum of money from the woman, he worked for, as a handy man. Without giving any reason for the killing he pleaded guilty. Despite his wealth, travels overseas and expensive life style he was not able to find a friend. He outwardly appeared odd, eccentric and devoid of social skills. In retrospect there were many casual statements he made with display of dangerous behaviour: could have alerted his health professionals to take action.

With these fatal consequences, mental health professionals must learn to refine their skills in recognising, the potential perpetrator with callous, insensitive and psychopathic tendencies. Some of the studies suggest that around 40% had some form of prior mental health contact. Lone attackers have high level of psychotic and non-psychotic disorders.

They are largely social isolates and believe in being victimised and rejected. Commonest diagnosis is depression though 10-15% of these killers probably had psychotic disorder (Gills P, et al. 2017).

Threats are the expressed intentions of those, who have history of self-harm, substance abuse, and anti social behaviour. They are distressed and disturbed people who cannot find a way out of their current dilemma and have considered suicide. However the enactment depends on individual commitment, level of preoccupation, plausibility, planning and preparation (Warren L J, et al. 2014).

Engaging the person in treatment both voluntarily and under the Mental Health Act may be challenging.

The Queensland Fixated Threat Assessment Centre (QFTAC): Established in Brisbane in 2013 in preparation of G20 Summit of 2014; a premium forum for world economy. Modeled on Fixed Threat Assessment Centre in UK, it was collaborated between Intelligence, Counter terrorism, Major Events Command of Queensland Police and Forensic Mental Health Services of Queensland. The main purpose of this unit has been to safeguard, the major events by prior identification of mentally ill or otherwise dangerous people, and prevent any harmful outcome. Several studies have found that a lone person with intense fixation on an idiosyncratic cause, grievance or a public figure, poses a risk of serious harm. Fixated person refers to obsessive preoccupation pursued to, pathological degree.

Mentally ill people may be attracted to public gatherings for many reasons. They can be disorganised, intoxicated or acutely psychotic people who may have incorporated, delusional ideas in their distorted belief system. Among the curious people the more dangerous are: attention seekers with personality disorder usually known to the police. And last but not the least is the angry fixated person with possibly untreated mental illness seeking revenge, which may not exclude unrelated or innocent people. Most fixated-individuals, who engage in, violence, exhibit warning behaviour prior to the attack.

Human and animal studies suggest that testosterone may be involved in pathophysiology of aggressive and violent behaviour. Testosterone may increase aggressive behaviour in women and is associated with higher level of criminal violence in prison female population (Dabbs JM, et al. 2001). Possibly testosterone is involved in the neurobiology of homicide.

Potential risk factors for recidivism/re-offending have generally been identified as:

Being indigenous
Less than 25 years old at the time of their first offence
Diagnosis of substance abuse disorder
Diagnosis of antisocial personality disorder
Prior imprisonment
Previous convictions
and Unemployed

Forensic mental health system can provide successful treatment and rehabilitation of identified people

References

Dabbs JM, Riad JK, et al. 2001 Testosterone and ruthless homicide. Personality and individual Differences. 31: 599-603.

Foulds JA and Monasterio E. A public health catastrophe looms: The Australian and New Zealand prison crisis. ANZJP 2018; 52:1019-1020.

Gills P, Silver J, et al. (2017) Shooting alone: The pre-attack experience and behaviour of US solo mass murderers. Journal of Forensic Sciences 62: 710-714.

Warren L J, Mullen PE et al. 2014 Explicit threats of violence. International Handbook of Threats. New York. Oxford University Press.

GENDER-DYSHORIA

ACCEPTED AS NATURAL spectrum of human diversity, the concept of trans-gender, has expanded many folds from the times of Torah, Christian bible and Koran, proscribing cross-dressing as defiance to God. St Joan of Arc was executed in 1431 at the age of 19 years for cross-dressing.

Christine Jorjensen, became the face of twentieth century trans-sexuality, when she underwent gender reassignment surgery, being referred by renowned American sexologist Alfred Kinsley, to the endocrinologist Harry Benjamin, who was instrumental in the process of its recognition (Dr Finton Harte).

The trajectory and the gradual transition to present stage has been remarkable where World Professional Association for Transgender Health was created in 2011 and the Mardi Grass parade is listed as one of most popular and entertaining event in Australia.

There are continuing attempts to minimise the stigma of gender dysphoria as a psychiatric diagnostic term. Therefore there is preference to use gender incongruence as described in ICD-11.

Case Study

A, 68 years old, father of 3 adult children, and 2 grandchildren was self-referred. He worked as a TAFE (Technical and Further Education) teacher. He was trying to overcome the loss of his wife, whom he married at the age of 22 years He grew up in a close-knit family, including his 3 sisters. His bereavement following his wife's death was complicated by his preoccupation with wearing her clothes. He felt embarrassed to talk about it to anyone though he found difficult to contain his recurring thoughts and resulting anxiety. He requested for a referral to see me without discussing it with his general practitioner. As he was able to talk freely, he discussed his discomfort of living in a man's body. After a few more sessions I was convinced that it was not just part of his grief, to not let go of his wife, but indeed long standing suppressed emotion specially in earlier times when gender issues were slipped under the carpet. Towards the end of last century he started reading about more people, coming out of the closet, which gave him the strength to speak up, though his wife's death finally liberated him. I suggested that he gradually discusses general gender issues with his family before sharing his feminine thoughts. The next stage was to gradually include female attire starting from less obvious items like jewellery, longer hair and clothing. He needed to change his name and get his social network to accept it.

Upon his revelation, there was furore in his family with rage. His sisters felt devastated and cried, as they were to lose their only brother. His children were concerned of its impact on their children. I was, at least partly blamed, by the family, for not dissuading him from this 'unnatural' conversion.

He had enough courage and strength by now to dismiss all the oppositions. He started to come for his visits fully dressed as a woman with appropriate make up and hairstyle. I referred him to an endocrinologist though neither of them felt the need for any hormone therapy.

He by now, with a female name started to feel that dressing up was not sufficient and she wanted gender reassignment surgery. Again with further assessment I referred her to a surgeon known for reconstruction surgery. She was happy with her new body and came to see me with a "thank you note". She told me that her recent appointment with the surgeon went well. "He asked me how is it going" and I told him "do you want a test drive".

She was readjusting to her new (transsexual) life as a woman, so I did not see much of her till one day I had an urgent call. She was angry wanting an immediate action. She went to women's restroom and was not allowed in. With some argument she was asked by the Council to provide a letter of her new identity. I faxed a letter to relieve her distress.

She formed a network of female friends "us girls", and felt that she did not have much in common with men, and that women have more fun, are more productive and lead meaningful life.

Her story is not, dissimilar to several high profile transgender people in the global community. It was very similar, to the American comedy show; 'Transparent' based on, its producer's experience, of her psychiatrist father's revelation at the age of 75 years that he was a transgender.

The modern liberated world with more individual freedom and respect for people's choices seems to be an ideal environment. Unfortunately it gets complicated if there is contamination by mental illness or dysfunctional personality, looking for alternate answers to their insoluble problems, within transgender life style.

Another transsexual couple I inherited was not as functional and pleasant as my previous patient. The identified male patient was seeking reassignment surgery to become a female in order to live with his/her partner in lesbian relationship. He was highly intelligent man with antisocial personality traits. A computer whiz: who claimed to get access to any personal data online, which he used as a threat against people he felt angry with, including doctors who did not comply with his wishes. One year while I was away overseas and he wanted to see me urgently, he returned at night, threw a stone on the large glass window facing the street, damaging the inside of our surgery. The next day it was discovered without any clue of the culprit. On my return when the couple came to see me he apologised for his angry outburst. Although the damage was repaired promptly we were relieved to know of the reason for the attack. Both our staff and myself were overjoyed when the couple announced that they had enough of Sydney and were moving to a quieter country town.

The biological and environmental determinants of gender identity, discordant with physical sex have long been debated. The current biological view endorses gender difference in the brain structures, which begins, to be established in utero: masculinization of the brain effected by testosterone together with gonadotrophins and direct genetic influences. Dissonance between brain and the body development has been demonstrated as a feature of trans-sexuality (Besser M, et al. 2006).

There has been long running argument in favour of same sex marriage for its apparent positive mental health impact. However most of the studies have indicated that as much as it stabilises the relationship to some extent, similar to the heterosexual marriages, psychological health of homosexuals and bisexuals is, far worse than for the general population (A B S 2007). Australia's largest study, to explore the mental health of Australia's trans, including gender diverse and non-binary youth, highlighted the high rates of mental illness, with 52.5% of people currently diagnosed with depression, and 48.1% having attempted suicide at some stage (Telethon Institute).

Marriage is a complex psychosomatic synthesis of 2 people operating at biological and psychological levels. Same sex marriage is not a conjugal view of marriage but rather a model of companionship.

Despite increasing acceptance of gender variation, stigma and discrimination are slow to disappear.

In Australia, the estimated number of transgender self disclosed people are around 74,109-296,435 (0.3-1.2 %) and 2.4% are unsure of their gender. (Australian Demographic Statistics, 2017.)

This is a sizeable population to plan their safe treatment without bias. Hospitalisation for a transgender person has its own challenges when the community enforces gender role against the self-concept of the person. It may require respecting patient's wishes to identify with male or a female ward, even if it is the case where the person is waiting for gender reassignment surgery, and may not look like the gender of their future.

There are emerging complexities in managing childhood gender-dysphoria, as there are increasing numbers of children, referred to gender clinics, both nationally and internationally.

The largest publicly funded Gender Clinic was established in 1975 in Melbourne with aim of improving the health and wellbeing of gender diverse group through individualised client centered trans-affirmative care. It averages about 250 new referrals each year.

There is lack of robust evidence for RANZCP to formulate any treatment guidelines. Therefore prescribing hormones or surgery in a young person is not advised for its long lasting adverse and irreversible effects on physical, emotional and cognitive health.

References

Australian Bureau of Statistics National survey of mental health and wellbeing: summary of results catalogue no. 4326.0, 2007 page 26.

Australian Bureau of Statistics.3101.0 – Australian Demographic Statistics, September 2017. http://www.abs.gov.au/AUSSTATS/ abs@ nsf/mf.

Besser M, Carr S, et al. Atypical gender development: A review. Int J Transgenderism 2006; 9: 29-55.

Dr Finton Harte. Gender-Dysphoria Clinic Melbourne.

Telethon Kids Institute Perth Western Australia Trans Pathways 2016: the mental health experiences and care pathways of trans young people.>transpathways@telethonkids.org.au<

DESTINY

SOME YEARS AGO, the dearth of psychiatrists in Australia, led to the criticism that public hospitals were loaded with difficult to treat patients, whilst private psychiatrists had the luxury of treating "worried well," from affluent areas of large cities. Although it may neither be selective nor intentional, was partly true by the nature of illness.

Case Study

An old patient of mine made an appointment, a few years after her discharge, when she was successfully treated for anxiety and depression. A 64 years old well educated retired lady of Indian descent, was sharing her home with her adult daughter, who also suffered from anxiety and panic attacks, and responded well to the medication and interpersonal psychotherapy under my care.

Her referral was for the symptoms of her poor sleep, diminishing confidence, irritability, recurring anxiety and lowered frustration threshold. She was unable to engage in her previously enjoyed activities. Psychiatry deals with life stories, and its biological, emotional, and social impact in the form of symptomatology. Every thought and emotion generates reaction in our brain, mind and body. She was generally a highly functioning healthy woman, till her husband's death, when she suffered from depression and recovered well. This was more reason for me to listen to her.

She informed me, that her daughter had met a young man of her choice, and was planning to marry. This was not her issue, as she was waiting for it to happen, and liked her future son in law. During their second or third meeting, enquiring about his family, she was stunned and speechless.

As a 16 years old school girl, she fell in love with this 19 years old boy, soon after he joined Indian Air Force, where her father occupied a senior position. Love flourished, much to her parents' disapproval. After over a year, her father was transferred to another city. The teenage lovers corresponded through letters, which suddenly stopped, and she believed that it was her mother, who intercepted the letters and may have warned him against it. She was heart broken though moved on and married a man of her parents' choice. She called it destiny that with billions of people in the world, her daughter chose the son of her first love. Her anxiety started to escalate with the thought of meeting him after 5 decades, and that too, with his wife. She was unsure, if she will be feelings rage, regret, sadness or happiness. I suggested that she writes to him, though it may be extremely difficult. She was worried about his wife's reaction. After musing over it for a few days gathering courage, she decided to write a letter, hoping that it will remain a secret between the two.

It was a story, which struck a chord in me, giving me a plot for one of my unfinished stories, which I have been writing for many years as a hobby.

Back to, my patient. I was invited to the wedding, and I felt just as curious to see them together. She later told me that she was pleased with her controlled emotions, and their formal interactions, though she would have liked to know the reasons for their broken relationship. I did not see her after the wedding though her daughter and son in law kept in contact.

Psychiatry has proven yet again that mutual lessons are bidirectional in therapy, not only benefitting the patient, but providing a great opportunity for the therapist to grow, as well.

THE FATAL ATTRACTION

Case Study

I STARTED SEEING THIS 51 years old woman with symptoms of anxiety, almost to the level of panic attacks. She was living with her husband, and had 2 grown up children living overseas. She worked in an administrative job, which she enjoyed. Her anxiety commenced over 6 months ago, and she experienced her first panic attack a month before our consultation. Although she was able to control it by distraction and going for short walk, it was starting to affect her work.

She was well connected with her family, as well as socially. She described her marriage as stable, though stale. She had no previous or family history of any mental health issue. We settled for using benzodiazepine in situations of acute distress, and 25 mg of sertraline in addition to CBT. As the therapy progressed I learnt about the source of her anxiety and panic, which she did not think was significant enough for reporting.

For replacing her carpet, she hired a man from the local retailer. She felt irresistibly attracted to this man, and they started to see each other about the time, when her anxiety started. As her lover started to expect more commitment, she started her first panic attack.

A man aged 53 years was referred to see me a couple of months after I saw the aforementioned patient. He was wondering if he had adult

ADHD. He was unable to concentrate, felt generally restless, had poor sleep and diminished appetite though did not feel depressed. He worked in city and commuted the distance of nearly 60 Km each day by train.

He did not have any previous or family history of either ADHD or anxiety. He shared with me: his preoccupation with a woman, he met on the train and fell in love with. The relationship was maintained for 8 months, when the woman had compelling reasons to move interstate. He was devastated and decided to visit her, in her new home a month after her departure. He felt the major setback with the lukewarm reception he got, and felt the relationship was over. He felt sad for losing the joy of being in love, and guilty for cheating on his wife, when his symptoms began.

Both the woman and the man had the same surname but it was a common one, so initially it went unnoticed in my mind. However they continued to see me on different days, before some similarities in their story started to surface, which one-day alerted me, to look for their address. And yes: they were the couple with fatal attraction and I was privy to both their stories, which completed the jigsaw puzzle. Although I felt a bit deceitful, could not reveal the secret of my apparent 'supersensitive' perception of their home situation. Working with the couple independently and without their awareness of it, gave me a huge therapeutic advantage, which I skilfully invested in their recovery, with the renewed insight that old was the gold.

MENTAL HEALTH OF DOCTORS

"A doctor is a student till his/her death, when he/she
fails to be a student he/she dies" Sir William Osler.

I CANNOT CLOSE THE book without addressing the burnout and
mental health issues of the doctors.

"Our health system would grind to a halt: were it not for the
altruism of health professionals, including doctors" (S. Leeder).

Providing the caring service, without concern about reward-still
ranks highly on the scale of what motivates a doctor in to the field and
remain there.

Doctor's work can be as stimulating and fulfilling, as it can be
stressful and demanding with psychological distress, anxiety and
depression.

In 2013 Beyond Blue National Mental Health Survey of Doctors
specially, females and Medical students reported significantly higher
rates of psychological distress, (9.2 percent vs. 3.1 percent) compared to
general population. It was attributed to high performance expectations,
associated with medical curriculum, intensive workload, financial
stress and sleep deprivation. In another Australian study 44 percent of
medical students were psychologically distressed and only 10 percent
have been diagnosed or treated for mental health problems (Leahy CM,
et al.2010).

At the global level, 195 studies from 47 countries, quantified that about 30 percent of respondents screened positive for symptoms or a diagnosis of depression and anxiety and 11 percent reported suicidal thoughts (Rotenstein, et al 2016). It was two to five times higher than in the age matched general population.

Lifetime prevalence of substance abuse in Australian doctors has been estimated 8 percent (Wile C, et al. 2011).

Psychiatrists and psychiatric residents abuse more benzodiazepines, than emergency physicians and surgeons.

Medicine is one of the longest professional courses demanding utmost dedication and commitment. Training pathway towards specialisation is a long haul, taking at least 6 years of primetime of one's life. The average age of trainees at completion of training was 37 years, which must accommodate the personal responsibilities of child bearing and rearing. The overload between work and home is predictor of depression in doctors (Nash L. 2015).

The depression is largely attributable to fear of litigation, fear of making mistakes, long working hours, and quantity and level of responsibility. There are misgivings and unrealistic expectations, like doctors are immune to the normal range of human-conflicts, problems, vulnerabilities and illnesses. Strong work identity equates illness to incompetence, and thereby threat to self-esteem.

Sleep remains a crucial issue for doctors with 24 hours of service alert. Sleep is an active biological state that fulfills essential restorative function for both mind and body. Insufficient or poor quality of sleep, have been associated with physical and mental health problems. It impacts on cognitive performance and has a bidirectional link with autonomic and immune systems

Working as a psychiatrist can contribute to the experiences of burnout and compassion fatigue; however psychiatrists also have distinct vulnerability to vicarious trauma that occurs in, clinical interactions (Isobel S, et al. 2018).

Burnout occurs in the situation of high demands and minimal support, which leads to emotional exhaustion and decreased sense of accomplishment (Kumar S. 2007).

Compassion fatigue is, reduced capacity or interest of the clinician, to be empathic, due to prolonged exposure to clinical work.

Work place stress activates neuroendocrine response, via hypothalamic pituitary adrenal axis. This results in cortisol release. Chronic activation of stress response, with chronic cortisol activation can increase risk of adverse physical and psychological health (Lupien SJ, et al. 2009).

Vicarious trauma occurs through the sustained empathy with another person who has experienced trauma. It can be compared with countertransference. Its impact is gradual and leaves lasting changes in the perception and views of the doctor, akin to their own life experiences. As traumatic experiences are common in psychiatric patients, its impact on the psychiatrist is inevitable albeit to varying degrees. Apathy, exhaustion, irritability, cynicism, and disillusionment are some of the significant symptoms.

The anterior insula, anterior cingulate cortex and inferior frontal cortex are active when people experience emotions. The same region gets activated, when one sees another person, experiencing an emotion; a process thought to be mediated via the mirror neuron system. Mirror neurons may be crucial in understanding how processing other's experiences in a clinical setting can result in replication of trauma in psychiatrist through vicarious trauma. People who are more empathic have greater activation of mirror neuron system (Rasmussen B, et al.2014)

Whether knowingly or not, a 'good' psychiatrist becomes wired to their patients, through empathic resonance, identifying and feeling their anxiety, distress and sadness, and subsequently becomes more susceptible to vicarious trauma. While the empathy can help the patient, the process itself begins to harm, the psychiatrist who are not, passive recipient. In response to the trauma of the other person, activation of neuroendocrine, autonomic and limbic system occurs as adaptive responses to the perceived mirrored threats. Repeated empathic engagement results in sustained and cumulative trauma responses. When the defence mechanism gets mobilised too frequently it may form the basis of burnout and compassion fatigue echoing the emotional numbing of post-traumatic stress responses.

Individual personality traits can influence susceptibility to vicarious trauma. The interpersonal relationships that underpin mental health care are bidirectional and complex (McCormack L et al. 2016).

As with many stress related conditions, mindfulness based activities, like daily meditation practices, can have measurable benefit on stress and modest effect, on subjective wellbeing. It is a Buddhist based practice, influenced by new wave of psychological therapies, like mindfulness–based cognitive, acceptance and commitment therapies, focusing on regulation of maladaptive cognitive and affective processes.

Being a doctor and becoming a patient is indeed challenging. The intellectualisation of medical training makes it, impersonal, kind of an illusion of immunity against illnesses. However when the doctor becomes ill, also becomes disillusioned with invincibility. The personality traits of perfectionism, and compulsiveness required for success can also cause, stress and related illnesses as well as delay in seeking help. Not only the illness is sensed as a failure, doctors are more concerned about its negative impact on their career, like restriction or disciplinary action by regulating authority.

Life is not static and ageing is inevitable. The most difficult transition of life's journey is: giving up your most cherished accomplishment and your most valuable investment, which has been your companion of last many decades: Medicine.

Retirement

Retirement: a relatively new concept of, 20th century is a, major life event. It should be the 'gold watch' you have worked for, with passion and dedication. It needs to be well prepared, exploiting your talents, dreams and skills outside medicine. Age brings wisdom, freedom and confidence and yet it opens the door to many unwanted concerns, like diminished physical, emotional and cognitive functions. Studies have demonstrated that age is a risk factor, for poor clinical outcome, litigation and underperformance.

Normal ageing related changes, impact on fluid intelligence; abilities such as novel or abstract problem solving capabilities, in addition to lower performance and processing speed, against crystallized intelligence; ability associated with learnt or acculturated knowledge. However, wisdom, resilience, empathy, optimism and compassion increases or remains unchanged with age.

Educational and occupational attainments, physical and social activities, medical and mental health status; all contribute to the resiliency of brain (Stern DT. 2006).

Seligman's theory of signature strength, argues that greater satisfaction is gained from, living a life that allows us to use, our unique skills and talents, crucial during ageing, when skills and talents change or evolve. To maximise positive and minimise negative affect, one needs to pursue realistic and emotionally satisfying goals, in selective domains (Peterson C, 2004).

There are personal as well as organisational preparations for which resources are available (The RACGP).

There is a lot to look forward to the old age, as only relatively healthy individuals will survive to older age band. The older generation may be more mentally healthy, than slightly younger generation and older people are likely to be more resilient, and accept the inevitability of ageing.

References

Isobel S, Angus-Lepan G. Neuro reciprocity and vicarious trauma in psychiatrists Australasian Psychiatry 2018. Vol 26 (4) 388-390.

Kumar S. Burnout in psychiatrists, World Psychiatry 2007; 6 186-189.

Leahy CM, Peterson RF, et al. Distress levels and self reported treatment rates for medicine, law, psychology and mechanical engineering tertiary students: cross sectional study. ANZJP2010; 44: 608-615.

Prof Stephen Leeder, Emeritus Professor, Public Health, University of Sydney Australian Medicine, 30. 17 October 15. 2018.

Lupien SJ, McEwen BS et al. Effects of stress throughout the lifespan on the brain, behaviour and cognition. Nat Rev Neurosc 2009; 10: 434-445.

McCormack L and Adams E. Therapist. Complex trauma and the medical model: Making meaning of vicarious distress from complex trauma in the inpatient setting. Traumatology 2016; 22: 192-202.

Nash L. From medical students to fellows: a focus on education and training Australasian Psychiatry 2015. Vol 23 (2) 109-111.

Peterson C, Seligman MEP. Character Strength and Virtues: A Handbook and Classifications. New York: Oxford University Press, 2004.

Rasmussen B, Bliss S 2014. Beneath the surface: An exploration of neurobiological alteration in therapist working with trauma. Smith Coll Stud Soc work, 2014: 84 332-349.

Rotenstein LS, Ramos MA, et al. (2016) Prevalence of depression, depressive symptoms and suicidal ideations among medical students: A systematic review and meta-analysis. JAMA 316: 2214-2236.

Stern DT. Measuring medical professionalism. New York: Oxford University Press, 2006.

The RACGP Closing a Medical Practice workbook. www. racgp.org. com/ your practice/business /management tool kit/module 13. 2012.

Wile C, Frei M et al. Doctors and medical students case managed by an Australian doctors health program: characteristics and outcome. Australian Psychiatry 2011; 19: 202-205.

CONCLUSION

The first half of the twentieth century was dominated by psychoanalysis, until deflected by drug revolution of the latter half. The gradual transition into more evidence based scientific knowledge, brought it closer to the zeitgeist of medical science.

The psychiatry of 21st century is a productive, scientific, exciting, dynamic, diverse and, enriching field, of medicine. Neuroscience of emotions, exploration of brain structures and functioning, genome mapping, and advances in pharmacogenomics, are fast changing the shape of clinical practice. The impact of, information technology, social media and e-mental health, have already signaled urbanisation and globalisation, disseminating uninhibited medical knowledge. Unfortunately even with this unprecedented advancement, therapeutic progress leaves a lot, to be desired.

The much needed and welcome share of biological science will hopefully, not deter the creative, artistic and talented individuals who have been traditionally attracted to psychiatry, more than any other discipline of medicine.

Disillusioned with psychiatry? Yes it is possible. There is great deal of time, resources and funding invested in mental health planning behind the doors, and proportionately much smaller piece of cake, gets in the hands of the patients, for whom the entire system exists. Productivity commission (2020) report basically says, that service models do not meet the needs of the patients, and the return on the investment at best, remains suboptimal. Maximum wastage: minimum gain?

I hope the future will focus on prevention, for the creation of healthier society. According to 2007 Australian National Survey of Mental Health and Well Being, 45% Australians reported having a mental disorder: sometime in their life. In 2012-2013 over AUD$ 9.5 billion or AUD$ 332 per person was spent on mental health related services in Australia (Australian Institute of Health and Welfare). This was updated by the Productivity commission in 2020 as $500 million a day and up-to 180 billion a year. Less than 1 percent (90.6 million) of Commonwealth funding was allocated to prevention.

To address the growing burden of mental illness, we need to address the wider mental health spectrum during the key developmental widows.

Prevention of mental disorders and maintaining mental health is a huge field: needing collaboration of multiple sectors and professionals. Apart from its biological roots it requires community environment, mental activity, work, social and economic environment, and personal attributes to minimise the stresses of living. Some of these will come from global, national or local policies at government levels.

Looking back at my transformation, which in the large part is attributable to the profound and privileged experience of being part of my patients' life, cannot be over-rated. The experience of human diversity, and the power of relationship with my patients, continued to shape me, into humility of giving more, and expecting less. Indeed these were the real education and teachings of life, and will remain the core of my professional world.

The obvious question you may ask is: what has changed in psychiatry over the 5 decades?

A study conducted by Royal College of psychiatrists in 2013 found that only a quarter of medical students and only about half of general public would feel uncomfortable sitting next to a psychiatrist at a party. Well, that is a progress to demystify, that we cannot read people's mind by just sitting next to them.

On completion of any journey and in handing over to the next generation, there should be hope, optimism, inspiration and stories of resilience inculcating the enthusiasm and excitement, for creating yet another world of growth. Looking at the massive transformation during my working life of over 5 decades: was indeed the most profound experience one can have. At times I did feel that I was trained for the last century and not for the technologically advanced world of a computer whiz. The safest way seemed like quiet diversion into retirement, and create my own world of stimulation and challenges, more zeitgeist of the period in which I grew up: like reading and writing, an enjoyable, and relatively stress free life.

Health is fragile and losses of life are inevitable: our patients are indeed heroic in dealing with the vicissitudes of life.

12 billion neurons, each, with up to 100,000 synapses: a miracle that most of us grow up relatively OK.

"A physician who fails to enter the body of a patient with a lamp of knowledge and understanding can never treat disease. He should first study all the factors including environment and others, which influence a patient's disease, and then prescribe treatment. It is more important to prevent the occurence of disease than to seek a cure"

(Maharishi Charak: The father of Indian Medicine 200 BC known for the oldest book of Ayurved Charak Samhita)

INDEX

All the proceeds of the book will be donated to the

ChildCan Cancer Foundation HPP
Cancer Hospital Gorakhpur UP

www.ingramcontent.com/pod-product-compliance
Lightning Source LLC
Chambersburg PA
CBHW021349210526
45463CB00001B/41